Chain Chain Change

Chain Chain Change

For Black Women Dealing with Physical and Emotional Abuse

Evelyn C. White

The Seal Press

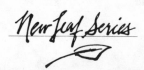

New Leaf Series

Grateful acknowledgment is made to the following for permission to reprint their copyrighted material:

Lyrics excerpted from "I Never Loved A Man (The Way I Love You)," words and music by Ronnie Shannon. Copyright © Pronto Music & 14th Hour Music. Reprinted by permission. All rights reserved.

Excerpt from "Weekend Glory" from *Shaker, Why Don't You Sing?* by Maya Angelou. Copyright © 1983 by Maya Angelou. Reprinted by permission of Random House, Inc.

Excerpt from *For Colored Girls Who Have Considered Suicide When the Rainbow Is Enuf* by Ntozake Shange. Copyright © 1975, 1976, 1977 by Ntozake Shange. Reprinted by permission of Macmillan Publishing Company.

Excerpt from *Movement in Black*. Copyright © 1978 by Pat Parker. Reprinted by permission of The Crossing Press.

"I Used To Think" by Chirlane McCray. Copyright © 1979 by Chirlane McCray. First published in *Conditions Five*, 1979. Reprinted in *Home Girls*, Kitchen Table: Women of Color Press, 1983. Reprinted by permission of the author.

Library of Congress Cataloging-in-Publication Data
White, Evelyn C., 1954-
    Chain, chain, change.
    Bibliography: p.
    1. Wife abuse—United States. 2. Family violence—United States. 3. Afro-American women. I. Title.
HV6626.W48 1985   362.8'3   85-18329
ISBN 0-931188-25-3

Printed in the United States of America

First edition, September 1985

10 9 8 7 6 5 4 3 2

Text design: Barbara Wilson
Cover design: Rachel da Silva
Composition: Accent & Alphabet, Seattle

Acknowledgements

In addition to many well-known activists in the domestic violence field, women in professions that range from bartender to ordained minister assisted me with this book. Through their comments and suggestions, each one made a contribution to the empowerment of abused black women. For practical and emotional support that has enriched this book as well as my spirit, I wish to thank: Dr. Trissa Baden, Sylvia Bogle, Julia Boyd, Maryviolet Burns, Faith Conlon, Susan Crane, Ann D'Antonio, Rachel da Silva, Barbara Daniels, Addie Rose Dunlap, P. Catlin Fullwood, Anne Ganley, Kathy Jones, Patricia Kalafus, Carolyn Lasar, Marsha Leslie, Jackie Moorey, Cara Newoman, Ginny NiCarthy, Renee Perry, Beth Richie-Bush, C. J. Smith, Lydia Swann, Joanne Tulonen, Dr. Joan Yager, and the many courageous abused black women who shared their experiences with me.

I am exceedingly grateful for the guidance, support and infinite patience of my editor Barbara Wilson. After working with her on various projects for six years, I can honestly say that Barbara understands the craft of writing better than anyone I know. I am proud to call her a colleague and a friend.

I thank my family Andrew Jr., Antoine, Angelo and Phyllis White for their strength and courage during a tragic time in our lives. They help me remember that it is not what I have lost, but what I have left.

To Linda Tillery I am so thankful for songs that will always touch my heart.

And finally, this book was graced by the warmth, laughter and generosity of Ann Hagedorn, whose friendship is my Pulitzer Prize.

Contents

*To the memory of Diedra Lynette Henry
and Lupe Duran White*

Introduction

About ten years ago, a black woman left her husband. The woman, a singer, had travelled all over the world with him, stayed in luxurious hotels and to all observers seemed to live a glamorous and exciting life. But in reality, this woman was being abused by her husband. For nearly twenty years she had lived under his complete domination and control, never knowing when she might be threatened or physically assaulted. One night after suffering another of his beatings, the woman decided she'd taken enough abuse. With thirty-six cents she walked out on him and started a new life.

That woman was Tina Turner. Today she is a Grammy Award winner and one of the most successful and respected singers in the music business.

If you've been involved with a violent partner for a long time, or seem to end up in one abusive relationship after another, you might think that it's all your fault or that you're just unlucky when it comes to love. Neither is true. Like Tina Turner, you haven't done anything to make your partner abuse you, nor is it your "luck" that's the problem. There are many traditions that support violence against women. The abuse you are suffering is also being experienced by many other women all over the world.

Unlike earlier times, domestic violence is no longer considered just a "family matter"—something to be solved or just endured by women like yourself behind closed doors. It is now recognized and treated as a serious social problem that is rooted in the acceptance of male dominance over women. Many people of all races are working to increase public awareness of domestic violence and to change the systems that contribute to your abuse. This book is one such effort.

In this book you will find descriptions of abusive behavior that will help you identify exactly what is happening to you. Once you understand how little shoves can lead to more serious injuries, you're likely to respond differently the next time your partner says he "didn't mean to hurt you."

You'll find information on the cultural traditions that have oppressed women in the first chapter of this book, as well as a discussion of the characteristics of abusive men and abused women. Reading this section will help you understand the pressures on both you and your partner to fulfill certain sex-role stereotypes.

In Chapter 2 you'll read about your experiences as a black woman in a society that is both sexist and racist. You'll learn about cultural images and expectations that keep you feeling like "the mule of the world," even when you know you're looking and feeling your best. Because silence will not protect us, the importance of talking about domestic violence and other problems in the black community is also discussed in this chapter. The process may not be easy, but it is the only way to work toward positive change.

There is also a chapter about the effects of domestic violence on your children. Understanding the potential risks to your children and the negative messages they receive in a violent household can motivate you to make changes even if you stay with your partner.

Subsequent chapters will show you how the police, health professionals, attorneys, counselors, friends, family, shelters, support groups and the church can help you end the violence in your life. After thinking you've been all alone in a world of trouble for so long, you'll be surprised to find out how many people are willing and able to help you. Throughout these chapters you'll read the words of other abused black women who thought they simply had to take it, perhaps like you do now. You'll laugh with them, cry with them and, I hope, use them as role models.

In the final chapter, you'll again hear something that has been repeated throughout the book—that you deserve and can have a caring relationship. You'll be encouraged to ask others for help, but also to realize that you are the best resource for making your life free from abuse. You can learn to love your strengths, accept your weaknesses and embrace life as a flesh and blood human, not the stereotypical strong black woman.

This book is for you, the black woman who wants to do something to change her life. It is also for individuals in the legal, law enforcement, medical, educational, religious and social service professions who attempt to assist you. Maybe you've heard about a police officer, minister or teacher in your community who is not as supportive of abused women as you feel he or she could be. Consider suggesting they read a copy of this book. It can help them be more responsive to your needs.

The social pressures that contribute to domestic violence affect men and women of all sexual orientations. If you are a black lesbian involved in an abusive relationship, this book can help you.

It is indeed my sincere hope that this book provides comfort and understanding for abused black women of all ages, incomes and backgrounds. The more it does so, the less pain I'll feel about a cherished childhood friend who will not benefit from this book at all.

"Everyone says he's crazy, but I'm not afraid," were the last words she ever said to me. This book will have no impact on the bright-eyed black girl with whom I jumped double-dutch, swapped penny candy and giggled hysterically through the night. It cannot bring back her innocence or the dreams for a future she didn't live long enough to realize. This book is too late to save the loving spirit of one black woman, but I hope it comes in time to protect the preciousness of many others.

Are You Abused?

Physical Abuse

Does your partner:

- ~~Hit, slap, punch, shove~~, bite, cut, choke, kick, burn or spit on you?
- Throw objects at or restrain you?
- Threaten or hurt you with an object or deadly weapon (a gun, knife, baseball bat, brick, chain, hammer, scissors, rope, belt buckle, extension cord, branch, bottle, acid, bleach or scalding water)?
- Abandon you or lock you out of the house?
- Neglect you when you are sick or pregnant?
- Endanger you or your children through reckless driving?
- Threaten or attempt to drown you?

Emotional Abuse

Does your partner consistently say or do things that shame, embarrass, ridicule or insult you? Has he said:

- You're stupid, filthy, lazy, nasty, silly, etc.
- You're fat, black and ugly.
- You can't do anything right.
- You'll never get a job.
- You're an unfit mother.
- You don't deserve anything.
- Who'd want you?

Does he:

- Withhold affection to punish you?
- Threaten to hurt you or your children?
- Forbid you to work, handle your own money, make decisions or socialize with your friends?
- Refuse to provide sexually, emotionally or economically for you?
- Force you to sign over property or give him your personal possessions?
- Tell you about his affairs?
- Accuse you of having affairs?
- Undermine your sense of power or confidence?
- Manipulate you with lies, contradictions or promises?

Sexual Abuse

Does your partner:
- Force you to have sex when you don't want to?
- Force you to perform sexual acts you don't like?
- Criticize your sexual performance?
- Deny you sex?
- Force you to have sex with or to watch others?
- Threaten to hurt you if you don't desire sex?
- Commit sexual acts that you consider sadistic?

Destructive Acts

Does your partner:
- Break furniture, flood rooms, ransack or dump garbage in your house?
- Slash tires, break windows, steal, tamper with parts or put foreign substances in the gas tank of your car?
- Kill pets to punish or frighten you?
- Destroy clothing, jewelry, family photos or other personal items that he knows are important to you?

Chapter One
What Is Domestic Violence?

You're no good heartbreaker, you're a liar and you're a cheat.
And I don't know why I let you do these things to me.

Soul singer Aretha Franklin was not the first, nor will she be the last black woman to sing about a troubled relationship. She did, however, in her recording of "I Never Loved A Man (The Way I Love You)," get to the heart of the matter in an especially meaningful way. Our intimate relationships can often be very complex and confusing, making it difficult for us to identify, understand or stop the abuse we may experience in our daily lives. If you answered "yes" to any of the questions on the previous pages, you are being abused.

The terms abuse, battering and domestic violence will be used throughout this book. For the most part, they can be used interchangeably to describe your involvement with a partner* who hurts you physically or emotionally. However, there are some subtle differences in their meanings that can help you better understand exactly what is happening to you. This awareness can help you feel less confused and better prepared to explain your experiences when you seek assistance from the police, family members, shelter workers, counselors, attorneys, etc.

Battering means punching, hitting, striking — the actual physical act of one person beating another.

Abuse may include physical assault, but it also covers a wider range of hurtful behavior. Threats, insulting talk, sexual coercion and property destruction are all part of abuse.

---

* Like many women, you may not be legally married to the man who is abusing you. In this book the term "partner" will be used in reference to both married and unmarried couples.

Domestic violence is a general term used to describe the battering or abusive acts within an intimate relationship. For example, a shelter worker, legal advocate or counselor who helps battered women might say that s/he works in the field of domestic violence.

Physical abuse, emotional abuse, sexual abuse and destructive acts are all forms of domestic violence. Some forms of abuse are serious offenses that can be prosecuted; others are simply behavior that no one should have to put up with. Your partner has no more right to hit you, threaten you or destroy your personal possessions than does a stranger on the streets.

Physical Abuse

You may be wondering if your partner's shove or occasional slap really deserves to be called physical abuse. Maybe he pulls your hair, twists your arm or puts his hand over your mouth to get your attention. He may shadowbox you into a corner and not allow you to move. Perhaps he chases you around your house and then puts a hold on you until you say or do what he wants. Although his behavior may not seem like such a big deal compared to being punched in the face, kicked in the stomach, or cut with a knife, these "playful" actions can progress to more serious injuries. Physical abuse often begins with seemingly minor "love taps" or harmless "roughhousing." This behavior can eventually lead to cuts, abrasions, sprained backs, punctured eardrums, black eyes, broken bones and dislocated jaws. Women who are physically abused by their partners suffer crippling, blindness, miscarriage, loss of consciousness and eventual death. Many domestic disputes become murder statistics every year. Some men actually do beat their partners to death. Some women do fight back and perhaps shoot, stab, poison or set fire to the man who is abusing them. While a playful push or punch may seem harmless, your partner's behavior may eventually become more violent. **There is no excuse and no acceptable reason for your partner to ever be physically abusive to you.**

Emotional Abuse

It is possible to be hurt in a relationship even when there is no physical violence. Emotional abuse can be as damaging as a punch in the mouth or a slap in the face. Where there is emotional abuse, there is always the threat of physical assault.

The effects of emotional abuse often last longer than those of physical abuse. As Beverly said, "The bruises from his slaps would eventually heal and go away, but I'll never forget the awful things he said about the way I look, the way I cook, how I take care of the kids."

If your partner has been emotionally abusive toward you, you are likely to feel depressed, anxious, ashamed and powerless. You may believe that people don't like you. Although you'd like to change your life, you feel trapped in a confusing situation and very insecure. You may believe, as your partner has told you repeatedly, that you are unattractive, worthless, unable to survive on your own and that you bring your misery upon yourself. Worst of all, you may come to believe that all black men are like your partner and that all black women suffer as you do in their relationships. The truth is that his constant emotional abuse, in addition perhaps to physical abuse, has worn you down and caused you to feel badly about yourself. **You do not deserve to be emotionally abused by your partner. You have a right to a considerate and caring relationship.**

Sexual Abuse

Sexual matters can be very difficult and embarrassing to talk about. You may consider reporting physical abuse, emotional abuse, or property destruction, but never dream of telling anyone that your partner's sexual interactions with you are unpleasant, frightening or violent. Because of your attitudes about marriage or your general views about female sexuality, you may believe it is your duty to perform any sexual act your partner desires, even though you don't find it pleasurable.

Your partner may reinforce these feelings by telling you that your attitudes about sex are old-fashioned or that other women will participate in the sexual activities you won't. If you decide to seek professional help about this problem you may be told that no sexual act between consenting adults is "wrong" or be misunderstood because of stereotypes about the sexual behavior of black women.

Yet it is very important for you to control your body and express yourself freely in sex, the most intimate and vulnerable of acts. For if you feel demeaned, disrespected or violated in your sexual interactions, those negative feelings are very likely to influence how you feel about other aspects of your life. **You don't have to submit to sexual acts you don't like. You deserve warm and nurturing sexual experiences with your partner.**

Destructive Acts

Some men display their violent behavior by destroying objects or pets. These destructive acts may be their only demonstration of abusive behavior or they might also engage in other already described forms of abuse.

If you woke up one morning and discovered that someone had smashed all the windows in your car, you would no doubt report it to the police. You'd probably feel you had been the victim of a destructive, criminal act.

If your partner damages your car, your house or kills your pet, he is committing the same type of crime as the stranger who smashed your car windows. If he intentionally damages items that belong to you as a form of punishment, he is abusing you. He may say, "Look at what you made me do," after destroying a gift he has given you, but you are not responsible for his behavior. **You do not deserve, nor do you have to be the victim of destructive acts by your partner.**

Domestic Violence —
Here, There and Everywhere

Your feelings of shame and fear and your isolation from other abused women may cause you to believe that every woman has a loving and nurturing partner except you. In fact, the abuse of women has been accepted throughout history and exists in all societies. In every major culture of the world there has been and is legal and cultural support for words and actions that keep women physically, emotionally and economically subordinate to men.

Although it was romanticized as a symbol of gentility, the ancient Chinese practice of binding women's feet is best understood by the old Chinese proverb: "Feet are bound, not to make them beautiful as a curved bow, but to restrain women when they go outdoors."

Menstruation, clearly one of the most natural and organic symbols of womanhood, has been considered taboo and unclean among many peoples of the world. Early Hindus believed that, "The wisdom, the energy, the strength, the right and the vitality of a man utterly perish when he approaches a menstruating woman."

Among the Fanti people of Ghana, if a woman was disowned by her family, her children were too because "children follow the mother's condition." However, if a man was disowned, his status alone was affected.[1]

Like these cultural traditions, the physical abuse of women has been taken for granted universally as part of the natural order of male dominance over women. The Russians said: "A wife may love a husband who never beats her, but she does not respect him." The Spanish: "Never hit your woman with the petal of the rose but with the thorny stem." The English: "A woman, a horse and a hickory tree, the more you beat 'em, the better they be."

Times have changed, but the underlying message of these proverbs still holds true today. A glance at any newspaper or television broadcast will confirm that violence, and especially violence against women, is widespread and accepted in the United States today. Most "action" shows on TV show men fighting with each other, but in fact it is women and children who are the most frequent targets of male violence. Authorities estimate that one out of three American women will be raped in their lifetime[2] and that one out of four girl children will be sexually molested before the age of eighteen.[3] This violence is a means of control, and is also directed against the poor, the elderly and the disabled. Violence against minorities also has a long history in this culture and continues today. In December, 1984, a white New York subway rider shot and wounded four black youths he said were trying to rob him. Many considered him a national hero.

Because violence surrounds us outside the home, many people find it easy to accept in the home as well. Teachers, social workers, police, ministers, doctors and neighbors have contributed, through their silence, to the systematic denial of the existence and severity of domestic violence. Although abused women come from all races, religions, classes and occupations, there is a tendency to label battering a class or race problem, and to claim that it only happens to other people. Yet FBI statistics indicate that a woman is beaten every thirty seconds in this country, and researchers in the field of domestic violence believe that no fewer than two million women are abused by their partners each year.[4] Physical punishment continues to be used to keep women in their place — whether that woman is the wife of a wealthy businessman and hides in the Lincoln Continental every Saturday night to avoid being beaten or the junior high school girl who is just starting to date a possessive older boy.

The Impact of Sex Roles

Rigidly defined sex roles, combined with historical traditions that oppress women, contribute to the social acceptance of your partner's abusive behavior. Some years ago, a group of therapists were asked to describe the healthy, mature male. Most characterized him as very aggressive, dominant, competitive and not likely to show his emotions.[5] Not only therapists, but many others in our society believe that strength, power and dominance are the hallmarks of masculinity.

These attitudes are reinforced by sayings like "it's a man's world," and "that's a man's job," that are repeated over and over through generations and that indeed, men are expected to live up to. For in this culture, educational, political, religious, recreational and military institutions all support and provide role models for masculinity that are aggressive and authoritative. Men are expected and encouraged to assert themselves with brute force if need be.

Even after the changes brought about by the recent women's movement, these attitudes and expectations about masculinity remain very strong. Rare is the parent (probably yourself included) who really expects a male child to wash dishes, vacuum or who encourages him to pursue a career as a nurse or librarian because those are considered "women's jobs" (and therefore have lower status and lower pay.) Equally rare is the parent who really expects a female child to take out the garbage, mow the lawn or to study physics and become an aerospace engineer. As girls and then as women, we are expected to be submissive, dependent, passive, indecisive, weak and emotional in this society.

As a result of this strict sex-role stereotyping, both men and women are constrained when they attempt to express their full range of emotions and abilities. A woman who demonstrates too many "masculine" characteristics is very likely to be called unfeminine, head-strong or a lesbian. A man who speaks softly or interacts with others unaggressively can be called effeminate or weak. If he enjoys or pursues a career in fashion, opera, music or dance he may be presumed homosexual because those professions emphasize grace, beauty and sensitivity.

It is almost impossible for men or women to live up to society's demanding requirements of them. Men cannot always be "manly," nor can women always be "ladylike." The pressure to conform to sex roles takes its toll on all of us. Most men, for instance, have not been taught how to express their "feminine" emotions. On the contrary, they have been told that they should never cry and that they should always fight back when challenged. They have not been allowed to express the helplessness, vulnerabilities, fears, feelings of pain and insecurity that all humans feel at some time. This inability to say "I hurt," or "I'm frightened," causes some men to cover up their vulnerabilities by carry-

ing out the masculine role to the extreme. Without permission or models
to express insecurity, dependency or low self-esteem, some men kick
instead of crying. Gloria, a black woman who married the captain of her
high school football team, illustrates the point with these comments
about her abusive partner:

> I think basically he does love the family, loves the children and
> cares about me. But he is so afraid of being judged by others.
> When he feels that his mother or the neighbors think he is not a
> good provider, it causes him great dissatisfaction. He may say
> he doesn't care what people think, but he looks for approval
> from everybody. I think it's because he never felt good enough
> as a child.

The particular circumstances that prompt their violence may vary.
However, many abusive men tend to be controlled and conflicted by the
sex role society expects them to fulfill. Although they may appear to be
"tough guys," many are often insecure, emotionally dependent, vulnerable and unable to deal with stress in a healthy or productive way.

How Does Battering Start and Continue?

Battering can begin at any time during a relationship and continue
throughout it. It can happen on your first date, on your wedding night,
after you get a job, after sad times or happy ones.

Some abused women report that the violence begins shortly after they
tell their partner they are pregnant and that the abuse continues while
they are carrying the child. They say that their partner often accuses
them of having sex with other men and demands proof that he is the
father of the child. The violence may be related to the man's jealousy or
dependence on the woman. He may be upset that he must begin to share
her with a child. Or perhaps he wants her to terminate the pregnancy
and spare him the pressures and responsibilities of providing for a child.
Because many abusive men hold traditional, conservative views, violence that results in miscarriage may be more acceptable to him than
abortion.

Your pregnancy can be one of the many excuses your partner may use
to rationalize his behavior against you. He may try to blame the behavior on his alcohol or drug abuse. Statistics do show that many men are
under the influence of alcohol or drugs when they become violent, but
these substances do not cause the abuse. Abusive men who have suc-
cessfully completed alcohol or drug treatment programs still batter and

some alcoholics/addicts never batter. It is not the substance that causes battering.

The "Cycle of Violence"

In her book, *The Battered Woman,* Dr. Lenore Walker describes the cyclical pattern of battering.[6] An awareness of this cycle can help you understand that you are not the cause of your partner's abuse and you cannot change it. His abusive behavior is something only he can change or learn how to control.

Tension-building is the first stage of the cycle. During this stage the man is irritable, uncommunicative and quick-tempered. He may claim to be upset about his job and have a short attention span. He breaks dishes, throws objects, has shouting fits, but then quickly apologizes. It is during this period that an abused woman may report feeling as though she were walking on eggs. She does everything she can to pacify or amuse her partner in hopes of preventing his violent outburst.

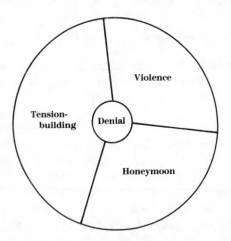

The tension increases and eventually rises, in the second stage of the cycle, to a physical or verbal explosion. A disagreement, traffic ticket, late meal, or misplaced car keys may send the batterer into a violent rage and he chooses to vent his anger and frustration by assaulting the person he is closest to. During this stage, an abused woman may be beaten for seemingly minor reasons or no apparent reason at all. It is not uncommon for the batterer to wake his partner from a sound sleep and begin an onslaught of verbal or physical abuse. One month after the

1982 war in the Falkland Islands, a woman reported that her husband beat her because he thought she had started it. Another had this to say, "At 2 o'clock in the morning he woke me up and demanded that I help him clean out the aquarium. I refused and he broke my nose."

Dr. Walker calls the third stage of the cycle the "honeymoon phase." The batterer becomes extremely loving, kind and apologetic for his abusive behavior. He seems to be remorseful and genuinely sorry that he has hurt the woman he loves. He makes promises to stop drinking, using drugs, gambling, worrying about his job, seeing other women, visiting his mother, hanging out with his friends, or whatever it is he believes is causing him to behave violently. The abused woman believes these promises because she doesn't want to be beaten again, nor lose what now appears to be a very caring partner and nurturing relationship. It is during this stage, when her partner brings her flowers, buys her gifts, takes her out to dinner and spends extra time with the children, that the abused woman's dreams of love and romance are fulfilled. She believes that her household has been magically transformed into the classic happy family, and that the two previous stages of the cycle will never happen again.

In reality, like the moon, the "honeymoon phase" wanes. The abused woman finds herself tiptoeing delicately around her partner as the tension-building stage starts again.

Changing Attitudes

The recognition of domestic violence as a deeply-rooted problem in our society has come from several sources, most notably the women's movement of the last fifteen years. Anti-rape organizers of the early 1970s first showed how women have been historically blamed for the brutal and violent crime of rape, and then silenced because of guilt and shame. Grassroots activists and, increasingly, social service professionals borrowed organizing and counseling techniques from the rape crisis movement to illustrate and address the similar plight of battered women. As public consciousness about sexism and its violent impact on all women's lives began to grow, shelters for battered women opened and social and legal reforms began to take place. With the anthem, "We will not be beaten," abused women and their supporters organized across the country.

Although it continues to face many cultural and economic challenges, the battered women's movement is here to stay. As an abused woman, you need not be silent or feel ashamed about the violence in your life any longer. There are many people working to change the forces that make your partner feel he has a right to hit you, as well as to change a society that supports violence of all kinds.

Being able to identify and understand (not accept) the physical, emotional, sexual abuse or destructive acts you suffer can help you feel less confused or responsible for your partner's behavior. It's not anything you've done, but rather sexist traditions and attitudes that perpetuate violence against women and children.

You may be thinking, "This is true for white people, but black views and experiences are different." You are right. As an abused black woman, you must deal with the effects of both woman-hatred and racial discrimination in our society. In the next chapter you'll find out how you have been helped and harmed by your experiences.

Chapter Two
The Psychology of Abuse

In addition to sexist and racist attitudes within the general society, an abused black woman has to deal with the complexity of her position within the black community. Understanding the special pressures on you and coming to grips with the sources of your joy and pain can put your relationship with an abusive partner in better perspective. This insight can help you to celebrate and protect black traditions that truly enrich you and to challenge those that contribute to your abuse.

Images and Expectations of Black Women

In 1928, black American writer and folklorist Zora Neale Hurston wrote an essay, "How It Feels To Be Colored Me." Today, nearly sixty years later, her words are still very much needed to help black women overcome the destructive images and unrealistic expectations that contribute to our physical and emotional abuse.

> I am not tragically colored. There is no great sorrow lurking behind my eyes. I do not mind at all. I do not belong to the sobbing school of Negrohood who hold that nature somehow has given them a lowdown dirty deal and whose feelings are all hurt about it. Even in the helter-skelter skirmish that is my life, I have seen that the world is to the strong regardless of a little pigmentation more or less. No, I do not weep at the world—I am too busy sharpening my oyster knife.[7]

The image of black women as long-suffering victims can keep us passive and confused about the abuse in our lives. Not only do we experience these feelings in our intimate relationships, but they impact our daily experiences as well.

In a contemporary parallel to Hurston's essay, noted black feminist scholar Barbara Smith points out, "... it is not something we have done that has heaped this psychic violence and material abuse upon us, but the very fact, that because of who we are, we are multiply oppressed."[8]

And who are we? Abolitionist Sojourner Truth, educator Mary McLeod Bethune, choreographer Katharine Dunham, playwright Lorraine Hansberry, opera singer Marian Anderson, Olympic runner Evelyn Ashford, politician Shirley Chisholm, activist Angela Davis and academician Barbara Jordan are all part of our black female heritage. Yet too often are the images of black women reduced to the big-bosomed slave "mammy" or the wigged and high-heeled streetwalker with equally stereotypical "evil," "domineering" and "bitchy" images in between.

The often repeated response that black women are honored within our communities is far too simplistic. It does not address the reality of the many hardships that go along with being black and female. For instance, according to the most recent FBI statistics, we are at a greater risk of being raped than any other group; fifty-seven percent of us raise our children alone; because of the job discrimination we suffer, our children can expect to spend over five years of their childhood as "have nots" compared to the average white child who will spend only ten months of his or her life in poverty.[9] We have been "honored" to endure these and other burdens that have often kept us from participating fully in life. And we have done so, not because we like being burdened, but because sexist and racist social systems have frequently given us little choice.

The images and expectations of black women are actually both *super*- and *sub*-human. This conflict has created many myths and stereotypes that cause confusion about our own identity and make us targets for abuse. Like Shug Avery in Alice Walker's *The Color Purple,* black women are considered wild—but also rigid and "proper." We are unattractive—but exotic, like Vanessa Williams, the first black Miss America. We are passive—but rabble-rousing like political activist Flo Kennedy. We are streetwise—but insipid like Prissy who "didn't know nothin' about birthin' no babies" in *Gone With the Wind*. We are considered evil, but self-sacrificing; stupid, but conniving; domineering while at the same time obedient to our men; and sexually inhibited, yet promiscuous. Covered by what is considered our seductively rich, but repulsive brown skin, black women are perceived as inviting but armored. Society finds it difficult to believe that we really need physical or emotional support like all women of all races.

The Tyranny of Color

All black people have, in fact, been damaged by the impact of color in this culture. A white Christmas or white-collar job are considered good and positive things whereas to be blacklisted, blackmailed or called the "black sheep of the family" have always had negative connotations. Although it may appear unimportant now that we are supposed to have achieved black pride, these images are constantly affirmed and reinforced within society. They have caused some black men, and indeed some black women to believe that white people, and therefore white women are "better" and more desirable than we are. Alice Walker writes in her essay "The Civil Rights Movement: What Good Was It?":

> My mother, a truly great woman who raised eight children of her own and half a dozen of the neighbors' without a single complaint, was convinced that she did not exist compared to "them." She subordinated her soul to theirs and became a faithful and timid supporter of the "Beautiful White People." Once she asked me, in a moment of vicarious pride and despair, if I didn't think "they" were "jest naturally smarter, prettier, better."[10]

These stereotypes about black women contribute to the confusion, inferiority and insecurity that you already feel because of the abuse in your life. These negative and often conflicting images may make you wonder who you really are and what is really expected of you from your partner and society.

Talking about these pressures with other black women can help you to define your identity and eliminate the many myths and stereotypes about black women. Make a list of all the black women you identify with and evaluate the parts of them you see in yourself. Likewise make a list of all the black women you do not like and look at what you find unappealing or threatening about them. If you could be any black woman in the world, who would you choose to be? Think about whether your choice is based on this woman's real contribution to enhancing the image and achievements of black women and black people, or if you'd like to be her because she is accepted by society and longed for by the average black man.

There are many passionate and celebratory aspects of our lives. Black women are as diverse in our ways of being as the rest of society. But this is easily forgotten, like many of our heroines, in the face of persistent messages that tell us our hair is too kinky, our behinds too wide and our tempers too quick.

Expressing your feelings about the complexity of your identity and the pain of your relationship is a healthy first step toward making you feel better about who you really are. If you don't feel comfortable talking to other black women about these issues, consider keeping a journal where you can write about your feelings and essentially talk to yourself. After talking about all that has kept you feeling down and out, black and blue, you'll find it much easier to nurture yourself and get in touch with all the things you really love about being a black woman. As black author Michelle Cliff writes, this "claiming of an identity" that you have been taught to despise, will help you understand and begin to challenge the abuse in your relationship and in your daily experiences. With time, you're likely to find yourself feeling like Maya Angelou in her poem "Weekend Glory":

> My life ain't heaven
> but it sure ain't hell.
> I'm not on top
> but I call it swell
> if I'm able to work
> and get paid right
> and have the luck to be Black
> on a Saturday night.

The Abused Woman — What's Love Got to Do With It?

Abused women have a tendency to put everyone's needs before their own. Because of our cultural history, this conditioning in black women is particularly strong. Perhaps more than others, an abused woman is likely to hold traditional views about love, romance and relationships. You make a commitment to your partner and even if you do not marry you have a big investment in the relationship. If married, you are likely to believe that your vows are sacred and expect a loving union with your partner for life. In exchange for fulfilling the traditional role of homemaker, you expect your partner to protect and provide for you physically, emotionally and economically. Abused women usually give above and beyond the call of duty to their relationships.

Thus when you are assaulted by the man you love, your beliefs and expectations about your relationship are shattered as well as your body.

Many abused women refer to the experience as having the rug pulled out from under their feet. There have probably been many good times in the relationship. Despite their violent behavior, abusive males can be loving toward their children and are sometimes greatly admired within their community. Consequently the abused woman faces conflicts both in her home and in her heart.

The entire nature of the relationship changes when your partner becomes violent. You believe that the violence is your fault—that it happens because you have failed to keep the children quiet or get the dinner on the table as soon as he comes home. Your self-blame is quickly reinforced by your partner, who as a batterer has learned to blame his violent behavior on you, the children, alcohol or job pressures.

In order to get things back on safe footing you are likely to work harder—to cook better meals, to always be ready when he comes to take you out for the evening, to give your partner more attention and to be more "feminine"—sweet, gentle and quiet. But it is your partner who is responsible for his behavior, however much he has conditioned you to believe it is your fault. It is important to realize that no amount of good cooking, love, attention or self-blame on your part will stop an abusive man from striking out when his tension level builds up. Until your partner learns how to deal with stress himself in a healthy way, he is likely to continue venting his frustrations on you.

It is not your responsibility to placate your partner or understand his excuses for his behavior, but to protect yourself from his violence and anger.

The Abusers

Because of institutionalized and individual racism in American society, black men, in particular, have experienced much of the power-lessness, low self-esteem, feelings of ineffectiveness and insecurity that characterize many abusive men. In *The Third Life of Grange Copeland*, Alice Walker writes with eloquent, insightful passion about the devastating effects of racism on a Southern black family. She explains, but by no mean excuses, the violent actions that some black men direct toward black women—the individuals *least* responsible for their suffering.

> His crushed pride, his battered ego, made him drive Mem away from schoolteaching. Her knowledge reflected badly on a husband who could scarcely read and write. It was his great ignorance that sent her into white homes as a domestic, his

need to bring her down to his level! It was his rage at himself, and his life and his world that made him beat her for an imaginary attraction she aroused in other men, crackers, although she was no party to any of it. His rage and his anger and his frustration ruled. His rage could and did blame everything, *everything* on her.[11]

Clearly the experiences of slavery, lynchings, segregation, imprisonment and daily urban living have taken their toll on black men. Historically viewed by whites as rapists, pimps, hustlers, superstuds and superathletes, black men are some of the most exploited and mistreated members of American society.

Many black men feel, for good reason, that they have no power and little impact on the culture at large. Thus they are more likely to demand that their partners and family members treat them like a man and show them respect. Any challenge, any question from his partner can be interpreted as yet another attempt to chip away at his already insecure and fragile sense of self. For black men know that regardless how hard they work, most will never become a part of the power structure of American society. And the few who do pay a price for their ''success'' with increased physical and mental stress.

The early deaths, high unemployment rate and excessive imprisonment of black men are directly related to racism in this society. In addition, racism has contributed to a statistic with far-reaching implications for relationships between black women and black men. According to a recent report from the NAACP Legal Defense and Education Fund, among blacks between the ages of twenty and twenty-four there are only forty-five ''marriageable'' males for every hundred females, largely because of unemployment and incarceration.[12] When one considers the existence of gay black men and those who choose to be involved with non-black women, the number of black men available for relationships with black women becomes even less. This situation is very significant in terms of the tensions that exist between black women and black men.

The average black man frequently struggles to provide his family with basic necessities. He looks for role models in the culture and finds, for the most part, athletes, entertainers, drug addicts, and armed robbers—the extreme successes and failures within society. The black man may decide that if nothing else, he will at least control what happens in his home and within his family. He may behave abusively because, like most men, he has not learned how to express his pain, frustration, lack of confidence and insecurity about his impotence in the world. But abusing those he loves only serves to make him feel worse, not better, about himself. For he has confirmed the racist stereotype about the violent nature of black men. He may come to believe that he deserves to be feared as much as society fears him.

The Black Woman's Response

Black women live in the same racist society that black men do and therefore cannot help but be sympathetic to what they suffer. We know that the black family has been damaged by slavery, lynchings and systematized social, economic and educational discrimination. Though we have surely been divided as black men and women, our mutual suffering has prevented us from completely turning our backs on each other.

Black women have been conditioned to repair the damage that has been done to black families because we feel it is our responsibility to keep the family together at all costs. We have been willing to let our children grow up with even imperfect role models because black men are scarce in our communities.

The importance of even the facade of stability in family life was recently emphasized very poignantly by fifty-one black children in Chicago. They took out a newspaper ad begging their absent fathers to show up so they could be loved and honored on Father's Day.[13] In addition to the hardships we will endure for our children, we do not personally wish to give up the tenderness and affection that even abusive men express some of the time. Black women, like all human beings, desire love, attention and protection.

However, because you are sensitive to the effects of racism and the victimization of black men, does *not* mean that you should continue to endure abuse from your partner. As poet Pat Parker writes,

> Brother
> I don't want to hear
> about
> how *my* real enemy
> is the system.
> i'm no genius,
> but i do know
> that system
> you hit me with
> is called
> a fist.

You do not have to become your partner's target because the bank didn't give him a loan. You do not have to become the scapegoat when the landlord raises the rent. And you do not have to become the punching bag because he can't afford to take the children to Disneyland.

Physical and emotional abuse are not acceptable demonstrations of black manhood, even though your partner, family or friends may try to make excuses for his behavior. Black men will *not* heal their wounded pride or regain a sense of dignity by abusing black women. It is important for you to hold your partner accountable for every injury he inflicts. By doing so you stop contributing to your own pain as well as to his self-destructiveness.

There are real pressures like poverty and discrimination that have contributed to the disruption of the black family over the last twenty years. But it is not until we begin to address these issues openly and take responsibility for what we can change within our families that we will move beyond our victimized status. For you, as an abused black woman, this means saying, "No," to the abusive behavior of a partner that threatens you or your children. Taking such action does not mean you want to emasculate him, but that you believe you have a right to a loving relationship. When your partner learns how to treat you with care and understanding, he'll feel better about himself and his abilities.

It is also important to remember, as Ashford and Simpson sing, that "love don't always make it right." Changing strong, culturally supported patterns of behavior may be a very long and difficult process for both you and your partner. On your own, you might not be strong enough to spend a special occasion like your birthday without him, even though you know he might become violent. Without some kind of help, he may not be able to take a walk, instead of hitting you, when he has to work extra hours.

Sometimes, the only solution for your self-protection is to leave your partner temporarily or, if need be, permanently.

Chapter Three
Staying or Leaving

The reasons women choose to stay in or to leave an abusive relationship are rarely ever clear-cut or simple. Some days you may be absolutely convinced that you will not stay with your partner another minute. Other days you may not be able to imagine a life without him. Living in an abusive situation distorts your views about what exactly the relationship represents to you. Understanding the emotional and practical issues involved in your abuse will help you develop a better strategy for your survival and self-protection, whether you decide to stay or leave.

Why Do You Stay?

In addition to your awareness of the black man's victimization, you probably stay with or return to your abusive partner out of fear. You know that he will physically harm you if you leave or act independently because he has done so before. He may have isolated you from family and friends so that you feel completely dependent upon him. Or you may have isolated yourself out of fear and shame that someone will discover you are in an abusive relationship and, in the "blame the victim" tradition, judge you a failure. You may want to protect your partner's job (your source of income) or your reputation in your community. You may believe, as he's told you, that you can't live without him, can't find anyone else who would tolerate a "stupid" and "worthless" woman like yourself. You may feel sorry for him because he has a drinking problem, was raised in an abusive household himself, or because he threatens to commit suicide if you leave.

> After he'd beaten me, he'd cry. He'd say he was sorry and it was just like he was a little boy. He'd be so scared I was going to leave him. You can't help but feel bad, that it's your fault when you see a big, strong man cry. Sometimes I really believed he'd kill himself if I left.

As an abused woman you may want the relationship you're in, but without the violence.

All of these factors may cause you to behave in ways that others view as crazy, stupid or self-destructive because they don't understand the particular dynamics of the cycle of violence or domestic violence.

You also stay in the relationship because you feel physically, emotionally and financially trapped by society's expectations of you. You know that people think you're stupid for staying in an abusive relationship, but will consider you a failure if you leave. It seems both your fault that you are beaten and your fault that you are too terrified or ashamed to ask for help. Your self-blame may be reinforced by your family, friends, police, clergy, and by legal, medical and mental health professionals who may try to make you feel that you are responsible for your abuse. Because of their lack of sensitivity and understanding of domestic violence they may give you no support for efforts to stop his violence or to leave the relationship.

Instead of acknowledging your survival skills and enormous ability to cope, society considers you weak and masochistic. As an abused woman, you are denied the compassion, forgiveness and understanding that you characteristically give to everyone but yourself. You feel shamed and disgraced by your experiences. But the disgrace is not yours. It belongs to the society that fails to protect, counsel and console you.

Advantages and Disadvantages of Staying in an Abusive Relationship

Many abused women look at their situation and decide that staying with their abusive partners is better than leaving. Because of the importance placed on having a man in our society, they believe that an abusive relationship is better than no relationship at all. You might also choose to stay in your relationship because you receive financial support from your partner, do not wish to disrupt your children's lives by moving, do not want to disclose the violence to family or friends, want the family to still be together when your partner finally reforms as he promises to do, or you believe that even a violent home is safer and less threatening than the outside world.

Because women are conditioned to make sacrifices and try to work things out, no matter what, you may avoid taking an objective look at the disadvantages of staying in an abusive relationship. Some of which can be as plain as the bruises on your body, others perhaps not so obvious. If your partner does not make efforts to change his behavior and you stay in the relationship, chances are that you will continue to suffer violence that may eventually lead to permanent injury or death. You will continue to have low self-esteem, little self-confidence and feel isolated from family members and friends. In order to cope with your daily existence, you may develop a drug or alcohol dependency. Your children will be exposed to violent behavior that may later cause them to become abusive or abused.

What You Can Do If You Stay

If you choose to stay in an abusive relationship, it does not mean that your situation is completely hopeless or that it is not possible to begin to make changes in your life. What it does mean, however, is that you and your children remain more vulnerable to violence that will become more frequent and more severe. Your partner's abusive behavior will not change unless he makes a commitment to changing it.

So if you stay, one of the best things you can do is to start taking measures that will protect you physically and emotionally from his abuse. You can begin to do this by finding out as much as possible about the situation you're choosing to remain in. By reading this book, you are already taking better care of yourself. You can find other books and articles about domestic violence at your local library or bookstore (see Resources). You can also begin to break through feelings of isolation if you talk with trusted friends and family members about the abuse in your life.

Because children often feel they are responsible for the arguments and fighting between their parents, it is very important that you explain (as best you can given their ages), that they are not the cause of the violence in your household. Explain to them that you are concerned about their safety and are trying to make things better for everyone.

You can begin to develop a safety plan to protect you and your children. Prepare a list of the phone numbers of people you can depend on in an emergency. Get an extra set of keys made for the car. Put away some cash to be used for a taxi or to buy bus tickets. Think about how much emergency clothing you would need for you and your children. Pack a small bag and put it away. If you develop a safety plan in advance, it will be easier to take action when you need to use it.

Although you are still in an abusive relationship you can begin to think about what it would be like to live independently. Imagine how you would earn money, where you would live and what kinds of friends you'd like to have. Find out about classes from a local community college. The Urban League or employment office may have information about job training programs. A church in your area might provide emergency assistance or space for battered women's support groups. Remember you can go to or form a battered women's support group while still in a relationship (See Chapter 7). Organizations like the YWCA and the local chapter of the National Organization for Women (NOW) will be able to give you information about shelters, counseling, prosecution, how to file for divorce, etc.

These are just some of the ways you can begin to think about and take steps toward a life and relationships without violence.

Leaving

Although it means freedom from your partner's violence, making the decision to leave your home will be hard. This is because any change, even a positive one, causes stress. You may feel as though you've failed or get down on yourself for uprooting your children. Even though he's hurt you physically and emotionally many times, you are likely to feel guilty for leaving a man who is insecure, feels inadequate and is dependent on you. As Beth Richie-Bush, co-chair of the National Coalition Against Domestic Violence Women of Color Task Force writes, a strong sense of racial loyalty also makes it harder for black women to leave an abusive relationship.

> Loyalty and devotion are enormous barriers to overcome. Black women be forewarned: there is already so much negative information about our families that a need to protect ourselves keeps us quiet. It is a painful, unsettling task to call attention to violence in our community.[14]

With all these things going through your head, you may lose sight of the real reason you are leaving. You would probably not be putting yourself and your children through such change were there not a very good reason for you to go. No doubt that reason is that you are deathly afraid — for your life. Remember his most violent blow and that there is a possibility you might not survive the next one. Keep in mind that the longer you stay in an abusive relationship, the clearer the message is to your partner that there is nothing wrong with his behavior or that you are "strong" enough to take it.

There are many options to consider after you have decided to leave an abusive relationship. Though the choices may seem very confusing and hard at that moment, you should be proud of yourself for putting the safety of you and your children first.

Depending on your circumstances and your finances, you might go to a battered women's shelter, a safe home (See Chapter 5), or to a motel, friend's house or the home of relatives or friends in other states. Perhaps a former employer or as in Brenda's case, a former school teacher, would be willing to help you.

> I guess I thought about school because of the children, I don't know. Anyway, I knew that my old fifth grade teacher was still teaching. It was hard, but I went there and told her I needed a place to stay because my husband was beating me. She remembered me and told me I could stay at her house as long as I needed to.

Regardless of where you go or for how long, you should take a packed bag of clothes and important documents such as birth certificates, bank books and medical records with you. Take the money you have stashed away or withdraw as much from an account as you'll need. You may have to borrow some money from an understanding friend or family member for an indefinite period of time.

If you have not already removed items of real or sentimental value such as jewelry, family photographs, your children's drawings, your high school year book, items your parents have given you, etc., do so before you leave your household. Your partner may destroy anything he thinks is important to you once he discovers you've left. One abused woman reported that she found the recipes she used to prepare her husband's favorite meals torn up and scattered all over the kitchen when she returned with the police to get more clothes.

Remember that it is not cruel, selfish or unfair for you to take what is rightfully yours. You should not feel guilty about taking anything that will insure that you and your children will be safe, clothed and have enough to eat for a while.

Avoid the temptation to tell anyone exactly when or where you're going unless you are absolutely sure that person is committed to your safety. For not only is your partner likely to try to find you through his own means, but he may badger and harass anyone he thinks has information about you. The best way to prevent a friend or relative from giving in to your partner's demands out of fear or sympathy is to make sure they don't know where you are. When you are settled and secure you can decide with whom you wish to share your whereabouts and future plans.

It's not easy, but it is possible to plan, save money, and develop the emotional stamina and confidence to leave your abusive partner. Hundreds of abused women have done it. You can do it, too.

Chapter Four
The Effects of Domestic Violence on Children

Children raised in abusive situations often feel both guilt and anger about the violence in their lives. They can think they are the cause of your partner's abuse. Since the family is the primary environment where we learn to relate to others, parents who fight in front of their children provide violent role models for them. Because they see it in the home, the message to children is that violence, humiliation and disrespect are to be expected in intimate relationships. As Joyce described it,

> One day in the shelter all the kids made drawings for their mothers. I was busy doing something and really not paying much attention to Monte who kept begging me to look at his drawing. Finally I looked at it. It was a picture of two people yelling ''shut up'' at each other.

Girls in violent homes may come to believe that all men are abusive and that women are naturally abused. Boys may learn that men have a right to batter women. Like their mothers, children raised in violent homes can come to know abuse as caring. They may repeat the pattern of violence by becoming abused or abusive adults. A black mother who had expressed great pain and bitterness about the violence in her childhood, still had this to say, ''It has been difficult not to be abusive with my own kids because that's the behavior I learned.''

According to a shelter worker who conducted interviews with incoming battered women, about forty-five percent of them said their children had been abused, too. The abuse is usually the physical fallout of actions directed toward the woman. However, children in violent homes can also be sexually abused, emotionally threatened and have their young lives put in jeopardy, as Yolanda revealed,

My husband never actually hit the kids, but he had a gun. He'd leave it lying around and then make comments about how "tragic" it would be if the gun accidentally went off or if one of the kids played with it and killed himself. I was terrified to leave the house. I didn't want to come home and discover my three-year-old had picked the gun up off the coffee table and blown his brains out.

Children often separate their parents during beatings and the psychological effect can be as damaging as physical injuries they might suffer. Said one abused mother,

My daughter's speech became impaired and her physical coordination got so bad that she was bumping into and tripping over everything in the apartment. She wasn't my child anymore. She was an old lady living with us trying to keep us from fighting.

Because of the constant upheaval in their lives, your children may have trouble with their schoolwork. They may even develop a fear of school if they've had to be the new kid in class each time leaving your partner has caused them to change schools. You may find that your child may not want to go to sleep at night or reverts to bed-wetting after a violent episode in the home.

Specialized programs with a professional can help children understand that what goes on between you and their father (or your partner) is not their fault. In specialized programs through the use of dolls and other toys, children are encouraged to express their feelings about the violent behavior they have seen or experienced and to release their feelings about it. They can also learn to control their own rage and to express it constructively.

You may believe that you are "protecting" your children by not talking about it, but the truth is that children need to understand as much as they can about domestic violence—most of all that it is not their fault. Some shelters have children's advocates on staff who conduct play therapy sessions along with coordinating other activities. Find out which ones in your area have advocates and whether children have to live in the shelter to participate in activities.

When you've decided to make some changes to end the violence in your life, consider talking to your child's teacher, school psychologist or social worker about your plans. If they have some understanding of the issues involved in domestic violence they may be able to offer suggestions that can help you and provide support. You might find out if they are familiar with domestic violence by asking them to recommend a book to you on the topic.

Children are powerless, vulnerable and completely dependent on adults to protect them. Children raised in violent homes see a world that is brutal, painful and often totally out of control. And yet, because it is the only world they know — one which is controlled in their eyes by their parents — they will naturally believe that what they see their parents do is right.

Through play therapy and/or honest explanations from you, your child can be taught to understand but not accept the violence in your home. Your child needs to realize that the violence is wrong and can be stopped. Perhaps while you are in a shelter, living with other abused women and their children, you can exchange ideas about effective ways to talk to children about domestic violence. In fact, it was while in the safety of a shelter support group that Betty found the courage to say that her child prompted her to leave an abusive partner.

> When I heard my five-year-old daughter saying "Stop hitting my mommy," the same thing I'd said twenty years ago when I was a kid, I knew it was time to get help. First it had been my mother, then me, my daughter was next in line. I'm here because I don't want my daughter to be battered. I need to change my life so hers can be better.

Research shows that with some type of counseling, most children are resilient enough to withstand the effects of domestic violence. All is not hopeless if your children have watched you be abused. Children need not repeat the learned pattern of abuse that disrupts their young lives. They can live happy, healthy and productive lives — free from abuse and violence.

Chapter Five
Emergency Response Agencies

There are helping professionals who can assist you in the process of ending the violence in your life. It doesn't cost a thing for you to call the police or go to a battered women's shelter if your partner is threatening to harm you. You can get the best service from the resources available to you if you understand their views and practices regarding abused women. It is possible to receive competent and compassionate service from police, health professionals and shelter workers that you might go to for help.

Police

The most immediate resource for an abused black woman in an emergency or life-threatening situation is the police.

What to Expect

Police attitudes about domestic violence have generally reflected those of the larger culture, and as the culture changes so do police attitudes. Some police officers believe that men have a right to hit women, that women "provoke" men into violent acts, that a man is "king of the castle," and that a woman who stays with an abusive man must "like" being beaten. Police are not immune to the sexist and racist ideas that pervade our society.

Two of the most common beliefs and the ones most likely to affect your interaction with the police as an abused black woman are 1) domestic violence is a private "family matter" in which the police shouldn't interfere and 2) violence is a "natural" part of black culture. Frances, a woman with a ten-year history of abuse from her husband recounted these kinds of experiences with the police:

They didn't give a damn, they just didn't care. They could see I was pregnant and that he had beaten me. But do you think they talked to me? They took him [batterer] outside for a while. I looked out the window and they were all just laughing and joking. The police were standing there admiring *his van*.

Asked if over the years black officers had been more sensitive and willing to help her than whites, she replied,

Black officers don't want to arrest another black man, because they know that it could just as easily be them that's going to jail. It's hard. I understand their position. But hell, understanding is not stopping me from getting beat.

Research indicates that responding to domestic violence calls is one of the leading causes of police injuries and deaths. For this reason some police officers dislike domestic violence complaints. Because they do not necessarily understand the battering cycle, some officers also develop poor attitudes about responding week after week to the same violent household where nothing ever changes and charges are never filed.

The role of the police in domestic violence situations can be a frustrating one for all concerned. However, the more you know about police perspectives (right or wrong), the better prepared you'll be when you call on them for help.

Changes

Thanks to activists within the battered women's and other feminist movements, police departments are making efforts to better address the many kinds of violence against women and children: rape, incest and domestic violence. Police officers nationwide are being trained to understand their racism, sexism, homophobia (fear and prejudice against gays and lesbians) and how to change their attitudes so they can more effectively do their work. Some are beginning to understand and respond sympathetically to abused women like Charlotte.

I told the officer I wanted to press charges and so he started escorting my husband out the door. As they were leaving my husband said to the kids, "See what your mother's doing to me." And the officer said, "Leave the kids out of it, you did it to yourself." And then my husband said, "She should quit saying what she says to me." The officer said, "I don't care

what she says man, you keep your hands to yourself.'' Then he
put him out the door and took him downtown. I was shocked.

Slowly but surely, police officers are beginning to realize that an act
which traumatizes children, leaves women mentally and physically
bruised, and that could ultimately result in their own injury or death, is
much more than a "family matter." With increased training and continued community pressure, police officers are gradually learning to ask
an abused woman if she has any injuries instead of "Who started the
fight?''; to suggest that she press charges instead of "kiss and make
up." They are learning to hold batterers accountable for breaking the
law.

Dealing with the Police

Though it is obviously difficult in an intense, life-threatening situation, you should try to remain as calm as possible when you call the
police. Explain that you are being assaulted and give your address
slowly and accurately. It is not important that the police know it is your
partner who is beating you. This may cause them to ignore the call or
respond more slowly because of their attitudes about domestic violence.
Let the police know immediately if there is a weapon involved. They
need to know where you are, that you believe you're in danger and need
emergency help.

It is impossible to predict how your partner will respond when you
call the police. Some men leave quickly, some become more abusive,
others wait calmly for the police to arrive so they can state their case.
The important things to remember are that 1) you have as much a right
to be protected from an abusive partner as you do from a violent
stranger on the streets, 2) police officers have a duty to do their jobs
regardless of personal attitudes they might have about domestic violence or black people, 3) the job of the police is to respond to and
prevent crime, and 4) domestic violence is a crime.

Arrest

Recent studies on domestic violence have shown that police arrests of
batterers can cut repeat battering in half.

The laws in your state will effect whether your partner is arrested for
assaulting you. A few states have a mandatory arrest law meaning the
police are legally bound to arrest your abuser within a certain time
period if there is evidence he has assaulted you. A mandatory arrest law

prevents the police from merely driving your partner around or suggesting that he take a walk after he has assaulted you until he "cools down." It has proven to be an effective tool for altering patterns of abuse.

In other states, the police have the option of making an arrest if they have "probable cause" (visible weapons, injuries, witnesses) to believe your partner has assaulted you. They are also likely to arrest him if he assaults you in their presence, if he attacks them, if he has violated a "no contact" or protection order (See Chapter 6), or if there are outstanding warrants for his arrest.

If the police do not arrest your partner, that does not mean that there is nothing they can do to help you. When responding to a domestic violence call, police can administer first aid to you, establish and maintain the peace, write a thorough report of the incident, give you information about counseling, housing, legal assistance, medical treatment, and transport you to a battered woman's shelter, medical facility or home of a relative or friend.

The police cannot force your partner to leave your house permanently, give you disputed money or property, settle child custody matters or force your partner to go into alcohol, drug or batterer's counseling.

The Police Report

It is very important that the police take an accurate and complete report of the incident between you and your partner. The police report can influence later decisions you might make about prosecution.

Describe the assault in detail and make sure the officers see your injuries. You may have to explain to them that bruises on blacks are not always as visible or look as dramatic as they do on white people. Tell the police if your partner threatened or actually used a weapon during the assault. They also need to know if he has violated probation, if there are outstanding warrants for his arrest and if he has a history of drug or alcohol abuse. Tell the police the names and the addresses of the people who witnessed your partner assault you. Give physical evidence of the assault such as torn clothing or broken household items to the police. After the police have finished taking the report, ask them for the case number of the report.

Should you choose to prosecute your partner for assaulting you, the police report will be an important factor in the case. In addition, it serves as an official document of his violent behavior. It shows your partner that you do not take his abuse lightly and that it is a serious crime.

Your partner may protest about police brutality against blacks or accuse you of "betraying" the race by calling them. There is no denying that the relationship between the police and the black community has been a problematic one. Historically, the police have been some of the worst offenders in contributing to or blatantly ignoring the violence in black communities. The most important thing to remember is that your safety is more important than any kind of racial loyalty. Police intervention will stop your partner's immediate violent actions against you.

Medical Help

If you have been seriously injured during an assault, the police should give you immediate assistance or call an aid car to take you to a medical facility. Unless you live in a remote, rural area, chances are there will be other black people in the emergency room. Contrary to certain beliefs, this is not because violence is a natural part of black people's lives. The stress of urban living often contributes to mental and physical problems for blacks that demand emergency medical treatment.

What to Do

When you arrive, let the admitting person know that you have been hurt in a domestic dispute and ask if there is anyone on staff who deals with battered women. Perhaps there is a black woman you can talk to, but don't feel discouraged if there is not. Describe your pain and injuries as completely as you can to the person who is treating you. Ask for photographs to be taken of your injuries. Because bruises on dark skin might not photograph very clearly, make sure that detailed notes are also taken.

If your batterer comes to the emergency room with you, you may be afraid to tell the truth about how you received your injuries. You may be afraid of what he might do to you later or what might happen to him. You can request that a staff person ask him to leave. Though you may be very confused, frightened or worried about him, remember that your safety and immediate treatment of the injuries *he* caused should come first. You have every right to explain what he has done to you without him being around.

After your immediate medical needs have been attended to and before you are released, be sure to ask for and write down the names of the emergency room staff members who have treated you. This should include doctors, nurses, social workers, clerks and any police officers who may have been called to the hospital if someone else brought you there. Later you should prepare a special envelope to keep all medical bills and receipts for medication or supplies you had to purchase as a result of your injuries. For instance you might need major dental work to replace lost teeth or a new pair of eyeglasses if your partner broke yours during the assault. Be sure to save the receipts for such items.

Even if your injuries do not require emergency medical treatment, they should be checked out as soon as possible after the incident. Though you may not see them or feel them, you could have internal injuries, as one abused woman found out.

> My wrist hurt a little bit after he beat me up, but I didn't think
> it was anything serious. But the days went by and it just didn't
> get better. Finally, it got so bad I could barely grip the brush to
> comb my daughter's hair. So I finally went to the doctor where
> I found out my wrist was actually broken.

It is important to go to the doctor because what you may think is just a sore, swollen limb may turn out to be a broken bone that needs to be set.

Visit your family doctor and explain that your injuries are a result of domestic violence. If you don't have a doctor, are embarrassed to talk about the abuse, or feel that you can't afford to see a doctor unless you are "really" sick, make an appointment at a local women's health clinic. You can usually find one by calling the YWCA, NOW or an agency in your community that assists women who have been raped. There is no guarantee, but the staff at a women's health clinic is likely to be more understanding of your attitudes and experiences as an abused black woman.

Abused black women may encounter both the myths and stereotypes about black women as well as those about all battered women when we seek medical help. These include: we like being beaten, we provoke our abuser, we are castrating bitches, sexually promiscuous, accustomed to violence and probably welfare mothers who don't care about our health until we are in crisis.

Given these attitudes, it is not surprising that we are sometimes reluctant to be treated by white health care workers, or to discuss our battering experiences with them. The American health care system, dominated as it is by white males, has historically been insensitive to our needs.

Remember, however, that you should never be made to feel ashamed, foolish or responsible for your abuse when you seek medical help. You are not to blame for your injuries and what you deserve is compassionate care, not unsympathetic lectures from health care professionals.

If you do not feel confident or comfortable enough to see someone by yourself, ask a trusted and assertive friend to accompany you. The friend can supply moral support and serve as a witness to your injuries and the type of medical treatment you were given. If you are reluctant to have bruised private parts of your body examined, your friend can take photographs of them before or after you are treated professionally.

Your physical health and safety are the most important reasons for you to seek medical treatment after your partner has assaulted you. Additionally, documented evidence of his abuse can help your case should you decide to prosecute. Your accumulation of medical evidence (no matter how small) may stop your partner from striking you if he thinks medical reports might be used later in court.

Shelters

''Nowhere to run to baby, nowhere to hide,'' describes the plight of an abused woman searching for shelter prior to the mid-1970s. There was simply no place to go. Fortunately, through the efforts of thousands of women, including many formerly battered ones, a much needed shelter network has developed over the past ten years.

There are an estimated 500–700 battered women's shelters across the country. In some cities, community residents also volunteer to house abused women and their children as part of a safe homes program. In Brooklyn, New York, for example, the Park Slope Safe Home Project not only houses women within the community, but it operates safe apartments where abused women can live on their own rent-free for up to a month as well. Though often forced to survive on minimal financial resources, battered women's shelters and safe home programs have been critical forces in saving and re-directing the course of many women's and children's lives.

Shelters are designed to insure the safety of the women and children who stay in them for a few days, a few weeks, or up to a month. Shelter locations are usually only known to staff and the local police. The most important reason for you to go to a battered women's shelter is that it provides safety and protection from the man who is abusing you. Family members or friends may encourage you to stay with your abusive partner (in the tradition of "strong black womanhood") or to forgive him and eventually go back. In a shelter, however, you will be supported by other abused women who want you to make the best decision you can that will eliminate the violence from your life. As Camille said,

> There was so much stress and pressure at home—from him and my friends to "work it out." So being at the shelter was like a vacation. The kids and I just didn't have to deal with that. I could finally think about what I wanted to do.

The daily routine in a shelter will vary depending on the policies it has. However, in almost all, the cooking, cleaning, childcare and other household duties will be shared by residents on a rotating schedule. You can expect house meetings, counseling sessions and group activities all designed to undo some of the damage of your partner's abuse and to help you make independent decisions about your future life.

The shelter will be staffed by women who can help you with questions about housing, jobs, counseling, education, health and childcare. In urban areas, there are often black women on shelter staffs, including some who may have been battered at one time themselves. These women will be at the shelter with you twenty-four hours a day to help you as best they can.

Just as important as the guidance you will receive from shelter staff is the confidence and knowledge you'll gain from living with other abused women who understand your situation because they have experienced it too.

> I really didn't want to go but being in the shelter really helped me a lot. Sure there were some personality problems and rules I didn't like. But I didn't get hit for not liking them and my son was not scared. The counselors allowed him to express his feelings openly. Besides for being safe, one of the most helpful things I learned in the shelter was how to deal with my anger when my son misbehaves.

Much of your isolation, your feeling that you are perhaps the only abused black woman in the world, will begin to change when you meet other black women like yourself. In the shelter you will also meet women of other races with different backgrounds and experiences from your own. You will meet women who have perhaps held down jobs, gone to school, found new apartments—all while being abused. You will learn from them that you are indeed capable of changing your life and doing things that your partner has told you you cannot do. Living with and sharing experiences with other abused women will show you that abuse does not only happen to black women, but to women from all walks of life. Most importantly, it will show you that support from other abused women can inspire you to change your life.

While you can learn much from the diversity of the shelter staff and residents, sharing living space with different kinds of people and following shelter rules may cause you some frustration. Because shelters are not immune to the racism that exists in society, some can be run in ways that are insensitive to the cultural needs or perspectives of black women. Sandra remembered this about her shelter experience:

> Some of the counselors can treat you like you're crazy or stupid. You can feel imprisoned or like a child. I'm a grown woman. And I'm going through enough as it is without having to go through stuff with counselors.

As an abused black woman, you may be reluctant to leave a familiar network of neighbors, family and friends to go live in a shelter with a group of people you don't know much about or have been taught to mistrust. If the shelter happens to be located in a white neighborhood you may feel vulnerable, visible and unprotected.

Although the extended family (family not bound by household limits) is indeed a part of our culture and tradition, you may not be accustomed to or like the communal style of living in shelters. You may find it uncomfortable to sleep in the same room, share bathrooms and change clothes in front of strangers from different races or ethnicities. Because of our history as domestic workers, you may take offense at the requirement that you cook meals, clean and perform childcare duties for other shelter residents, some of whom may be white. You may not understand why alcohol and non-prescription drugs are not allowed or why you will be forbidden to spank your child, as is the case in most shelters. You may not like the curfews or signing out systems that many shelters have to make sure residents are always accounted for. You may disagree with the rule that you can't even tell your best girlfriend the address of the shelter.

Although you may feel like they were made up specifically to oppress you, most shelter rules exist for a reason—to keep violent and potentially dangerous men away from the women and children they have abused. "If one woman tells her partner where the shelter is, it can affect the whole group," said a counselor. "Many women fear revenge from any man who comes near the shelter. It's contagious."

However, if the shelter has rules that you feel disregard your feelings or experiences as a black woman, do not be afraid to discuss it in a house meeting or with an individual staff member. You can use the experience to get back some of the sense of power your partner has driven out of you as well as to help foster the cultural sensitivity that will make shelters and other service agencies more responsive to the needs of black women. Talk up if you are made to feel uncomfortable about the kind of food you cook, the music you listen to or the way you comb your children's hair. A simple comment like, "I'd rather do yardwork or answer phones today instead of cooking because too much time in the kitchen makes me feel like a maid," will point out to other shelter residents that you are willing to do your fair share of chores, but not at the expense of your self-esteem.

You may feel uneasy speaking up for yourself because of your experiences with an abusive partner. Remember that though you may experience conflicts, communication problems, or blatant racist incidents while in the shelter, no one is going to batter you for expressing your feelings.

Some abused women, like Paula, report that they made friends for life while at a battered women's shelter.

> It just seemed like Diane and I had so much in common. I found out we'd even cussed out the same police officers. In the shelter we'd help each other out with the kids and trying to find apartments and just doing all the stuff that seems so hard unless there's somebody who understands. I eventually went to my mother's but Diane and I stayed in touch and we do to this day.

There are many different types of shelters. For instance, the Park Slope Safe Home Project, which was described earlier, is run by a group of women in that Brooklyn community. Shelters can also be run by church groups, the YWCA, the Salvation Army, women's organizations or the local city government.

You should check the telephone listings (often located at the front of the book with other emergency numbers) under "Battered" or "Abused Women" to find out about shelter services in your area. Your local police department or community crisis line should also be able to give you information about shelters. You can ask any of these people for the toll-free domestic violence hotline number that provides information about shelters throughout the country. You might want to write down all these numbers and put them in your address book.

After your safety, the greatest benefit of staying in a shelter is that you will meet other abused women like yourself. With their support, you can laugh, cry and begin to work toward ending the violence in your life.

Chapter Six

The Legal System

A general understanding of how women have been viewed within the legal system will help you feel less threatened and more in control when dealing with legal professionals about the violence in your life. With an understanding of some of its practices and traditions, you can make the system serve you better as an abused black woman.

Blacks and the Legal System

English common law, which America inherited when the country was founded, contributes to the tolerance of violence against women within our legal system today. Seventeenth century English common law held "by rule of thumb" that a man could beat a woman with a rod no thicker than his thumb. The routine beating of women went unchallenged because women were not considered human beings, but rather property. This tradition of male "ownership" and domination of others still exists in our culture today. For example, boats and cars are commonly referred to by the pronoun "she." The most devastating example, however, of people legally transformed into property, was the black American experience of slavery.

Through a combination of racist attitudes and the legal system, white males were able to rationalize and maintain their control over black people during slavery. Blacks, because of our dark skin, were viewed as savage, dangerous and naturally inferior to whites. Whites believed that slavery tempered the "heathen" tendencies of blacks and tamed what they believed to be our unrestrained sexuality. Because whites refused to believe that blacks were capable of loving or forming emotional bonds with each other, marriage between slaves was not legally binding.

These beliefs helped whites rationalize their cruel and systematic destruction of black families. By their thinking, since we couldn't love like other human beings, what did it matter if a child was torn from his/her mother and sold away? The following sentiment, expressed by a Southern writer in 1852, generally prevailed: "A slave has no more legal authority over his child than a cow over her calf." Black women were thus reduced to the level of domestic animals. Just as a brood mare could not be raped or abused, neither could a black woman.

Fortunately the official laws that permitted wife-beating and slavery no longer exist. But it would be naive to think that those sexist and racist attitudes don't still influence the American justice system. Blacks have learned through countless painful experiences that not all people are created equal and not everyone receives equal protection under the law.

Reasons to Use the Legal System

Though you may be reluctant to "bring down the law" on another black person, the legal system can protect you and help you feel less victimized by the man who is abusing you. If you were injured by a stranger, you would probably phone the police, report it and find out your legal options. Taking such action would make you feel more powerful and could possibly deter the stranger from assaulting someone else. You can look at the situation between you and an abusive partner in the same light. The laws that give you legal protection against a violent stranger also apply to the man who is abusing you. There is no question that black men have suffered discrimination at the hands of racist judges and attorneys. But the laws that protect you from domestic violence are not laws against black men. They are laws against crime.

There is always the possibility that a judge or attorney might make a racist comment or tell you to be a "better wife" should you use the legal system to stop the abuse in your life. On the other hand, there is the certainty that you will be abused again if you do not take some step toward letting your partner know that his behavior is unacceptable and indeed against the law. One option you might consider is filing for a protection order.

Protection Orders

A protection order is an official court document designed to prevent violence by one member of a household against another. Most states in the country have passed laws that make the order available to you. Although the filing procedures and fees may vary depending on where you live, you will usually not have to hire a lawyer to get a protection order. The charges for it are often minimal or can be waived if you have a low income. In some states the court can order your partner to repay you for the costs of obtaining a protection order.

A protection order prohibits your partner from threatening, striking or harassing you. Depending on state law, it can also protect and give you temporary custody of your children, order your partner out of your home and/or to enter a counseling program. If any part of the order is violated, your partner can be jailed, fined or both. The police have the responsibility to enforce your protection order.

How to Get a Protection Order

The process for obtaining a protection order usually involves filing forms and later testifying about your abuse before a judge in a court hearing. Your partner will be notified that you have filed for the order and also asked to attend the hearing. Hearing testimony from both of you will enable the judge to issue an order that is based on as much information as possible about your relationship.

Your state laws will determine how long your protection order is effective and the procedures you must follow if you decide to change or terminate it. You can find out specific guidelines about protection orders in your state by contacting a legal aid clinic, a battered women's shelter or the local police.

Other Legal Options

If you decide to take legal action, there are two separate and distinct legal systems that can provide assistance for you: criminal and civil. Criminal law involves crimes against the state such as assault, murder, rape, theft, property destruction and prostitution. Civil law involves disputes between private parties. This includes processes such as civil protection orders, divorce, child custody, support payments, property rights, malpractice, personal injury, etc.

If you decide to press charges against your abuser, you will enter the criminal justice system. If there is sufficient evidence that a crime has been committed, then a prosecutor for the state will begin proceedings free of charge, on your behalf. This is why it is very important that accurate and detailed police reports be taken. The description of injuries in the report, photographs, medical records, witness accounts, the presence of weapons and any previous history of violence in your relationship, will be critical factors in determining whether your partner is convicted of a crime and the type of sentence he receives.

Benefits of Prosecution

The purpose of prosecution is not to put batterers in jail or deny black men their "manhood," but rather to begin a process that helps stop violence in the home. In most states once charges are filed a "no contact" or protection order can be issued, preventing your partner from contacting you before the trial. This can give you time to think about your situation and make plans to improve your life without his menacing presence. If he is found guilty of abusing you, the order can be extended for a specified amount of time. Instead of jail time, the court can order that he complete batterer's and/or alcohol/drug counseling, pay for your medical treatment or damaged property, perform community service hours, pay court costs or serve probation. And of course the court can rule that he spend some time in jail, depending on the severity of your injuries and what kind of record your partner has.

The major benefit of prosecution is that it forces your partner to take responsibility for his abusive actions and begin working toward change. He may say you "made" him hit you, that you are putting him in jail, that you don't understand him and that the entire world is against him because he's a black male. The truth is that he is responsible for choosing violence when he is under stress and he must learn that violence is not acceptable behavior.

Prosecution serves several other important functions aside from forcing your partner to take responsibility for abusing you. Prosecution is a positive action that can raise your self-esteem and help you take control of your life. You begin to move out of the helpless "victim" role when you take the abusive situation out of his hands and into your own. The court process can help you begin to examine feelings about being abused that you may have repressed. Internalized feelings of anger, shame, guilt and self-hatred may begin to surface, enabling you to release them and heal. You may feel truly empowered because you have taken a step toward change. Regardless of the outcome, the trial can serve as a symbolic ending to your abuse. You will have shown your partner that you will no longer be passive and take his abuse. The prospect of standing in front of another judge may make him think twice before striking you again.

Civil Cases

The prosecutor will not be able to help you with divorce, support payments, or settling child custody/visitation rights because they are not criminal matters. For these legal problems you will need to hire a private civil attorney.

Choosing a Civil Attorney

Usually beginning at about $75 per hour, attorney's fees are expensive. So it is important to hire one who will be supportive of you as an abused black woman. It is easy to feel intimidated by an attorney's language or attitude. But remember you are paying the fee and therefore deserve to be treated professionally. If the attorney you hire ignores your request for explanations or to be regularly informed of the status of your case, then hire a new one. You don't have to give your money to someone who treats you like you don't have any sense.

It might be helpful to prepare a list of questions to determine if the attorney will be supportive of you. These are a few you might want to ask:

1. What services will I be charged for and when do you expect payment?

2. Have you ever helped an abused woman before?

3. Will you answer my questions even though they may seem irrelevant or unimportant to you?

4. Will you understand if I have to bring my children with me to your office on occasion?

5. Will you inform me if there are critical decisions that need to be made about my case?

The responses to these questions should give you a clear idea if your attorney is willing to give you competent and compassionate service.

Legal Aid, Lawyer Referral agencies, women's groups and black organizations like the Urban League are usually the best sources for information about low-cost private attorneys. If there is a major university in your city, it probably has a law school. Call the law school and ask if students run a legal clinic in the community. You can also find self-help legal materials in libraries and bookstores that explain how to do some legal procedures yourself.

Even an attorney who charges minimal fees ($35–60 per hour) will probably be asking for more money than your budget allows. It may seem unfair that you can't get help because you can't afford it. And because so many abused women need an attorney when they are in crisis, your sense of urgency and desperation may make the situation seem even more unfair. This is because many of us have been raised with the belief that lawyers uphold social morals, battle injustices and always help the "down and out." This is to some extent true. However, the legal profession is also a business — one in which women, minorities, the poor and disadvantaged are frequently left out. The best way to deal with this situation is to know from the beginning what you are up against financially. You may have to start saving up for your divorce as you would for college tuition or to purchase a new household item. Ask other women if they have hired attorneys who they felt were particularly helpful. Find out if you can set up payment plans with your attorney. A friend or family member who might not loan you money for other things might be happy to pay for legal assistance that will help you end the violence in your life.

It is not unusual to become very close to someone who is helping you with emotional issues like child custody and divorce. Your attorney will no doubt come to know many intimate details about your life. It is important to remember, however, that you have hired the attorney to provide you with supportive legal services, not to be your counselor or personal friend.

Avoid the temptation to make unnecessary personal phone calls (almost all attorneys charge for telephone consultation), or to seek non-legal advice from your attorney. If you contact your attorney too often for non-legal matters, you may get your feelings hurt as well as a bill for what you thought was just "friendly conversation." Remember the attorney has many other clients and is often in court most of the day. S/he may not be able to return your calls or see you should you drop by the office without an appointment. Your attorney has been trained and hired to give you legal assistance and, though concerned about you, may feel uncomfortable when asked to provide other kinds of advice. If you are feeling depressed, anxious, sad, or angry (all natural feelings) about an upcoming trial or life in general, a battered women's advocate or professional counselor can provide support for you.

Advocates

An advocate is a person who serves as an intermediary between abused women and the police, prosecutors, counselors, doctors, etc. The advocate is specially trained in the social and legal issues of domestic violence and will work with you to help make positive changes in your life. S/he will interview you and witnesses (though not usually your partner) about an abusive incident, gather medical records, photographs, explain procedures to you and may process paperwork such as "no contact" or protection orders.

You can ask the advocate to take you to a courtroom to familiarize you with the surroundings before your case comes up for trial. The advocate can help overworked prosecutors investigate and understand the specific details of your case and thus improve the chances that there will be a positive outcome for you at the trial. S/he may be able to make recommendations to the court about what methods of treatment (i.e. jail, batterer's counseling, fines) would make your partner take responsibility for his actions and stop abusing you.

An advocate can boost your morale and provide reassurance during the tense times before a trial (often four–six weeks), when there may be great pressure on you to return to your partner or to drop the charges that have been filed against him. Some prosecutors have "no-drop" policies to help take some of this pressure off abused women. Others believe that abused women should be allowed to drop the charges if they so decide, simply because they have been forbidden most of their lives to make independent choices or because they are truly terrified by what their partners have threatened to do if the case goes to trial. In any event, the advocate will be there to answer your questions and listen to your fears. As Jeanine said,

> I had times when I wanted to drop the charges. I'd talk to him and he'd say he was going to go to jail for sure this time. And what good would he be in jail if he couldn't work, is what I thought. He'd say he was trying to get in a drug program, trying to straighten up and it sounded convincing to me. Every-time I called and tried to drop the charges, the advocate wouldn't let me. Sometimes I even tried to disguise my voice. But she knew it was me and she'd explain why he was acting like he'd reformed. So I went ahead with the trial because I didn't have a choice. And I'm glad I didn't.

You can call your city prosecutor's office to find out if battered women's advocates are on staff. Advocates also work with shelters, police departments, hospitals and victims assistance programs. In addition to the prosecutor's office you might phone a shelter, rape crisis line, feminist organization, legal service agency or the social work department of a hospital to ask if there is an advocate to assist you.

What to Expect in the Courtroom

The laws of the city or state you live in and the specific circumstances of your case will determine how the trial proceeds. Your partner will have the option of choosing a bench trial (judge hears the evidence and decides the verdict) or a jury trial in which you may or may not have to testify. Sometimes prosecutors will attempt to work out a plea bargain with your partner's attorney because of the volume of domestic violence cases. In such an arrangement, your partner may plead guilty to simple assault instead of assault, for example, and not go ahead with a trial. You should be consulted by the prosecutor before such a decision is made. Your safety or personal wishes should not be disregarded just because there's a need to keep things moving in court.

If you do have to testify during the trial, you may want friends or family members to be present in the courtroom. Your abuser may have asked some of his acquaintances to come and their presence might be frightening or intimidating to you. Try to identify people in your life who will be supportive during what could be an unnerving process and ask them to come.

Your manner of dress, choice of words and attitude can reinforce or change stereotypes court officials or jurors might have about abused women. You can prepare for that by asking advice from friends who've been to court or an advocate. The most important thing to remember is to be honest in court. No matter what happens during the proceeding, you will feel good about yourself and appear to be a believable witness if you listen carefully, speak clearly, remain calm and simply tell the truth about what happened to you.

There are many reasons why you might feel reluctant to use the legal system to stop your partner from abusing you. You might fear retaliation, or that he might go to jail or lose his job. Perhaps you don't want your children to testify in court or feel that you will be ridiculed and intimated on the witness stand. You may simply not trust judges, juries and attorneys who have historically discriminated against black people. All of these feelings are legitimate, so do not be ashamed or afraid to express them. Simply remember that if you choose to use the legal system it does not mean you are a ''traitor'' to the race or that there will be no one to support you in your decision. You have every right to take control of your life and there are many people who are willing to help you.

Chapter Seven
Getting Support

After having your emergency needs attended to or taking legal action, you might find that you are still confused or frightened about the abuse in your life. Although the violence has stopped, you may be wondering if you'll ever feel like a "normal" human being or if you're able to become involved in another relationship. You can get in touch with your feelings and learn skills that will help you through the next stages of your life by seeing a professional counselor. Support groups, relatives, friends and your church can also be of help to you when you're feeling overwhelmed by your experiences as an abused woman.

Counseling

Because you can still get up and go to work every morning or get the kids off to school, you may feel that you are coping well with the abuse in your life. And you should feel proud of yourself for being able to function in a violent and unpredictable household. But you should also know that you do not have to carry the burden alone. There is nothing wrong with asking for help when you feel you can no longer cope. There are trained counselors who can help you deal with the effects of the physical and emotional abuse in your life.

All humans experience mild forms of depression at some point during their lives. The depression can usually be traced to a specific event and leaves after a short while. If, however, you are unable to sleep or find yourself feeling sad, hopeless, dejected, anxious or crying uncontrollably for extended periods of time, you may need professional help. This does not mean that you are crazy or that you are having a nervous breakdown. It simply means that you have been affected by the violence in your life and with good reason. You *would* be crazy if you thought you could be punched and degraded regularly, but come out unscathed.

Living with violence creates emotional problems that not even you and your mother or best girlfriend can sort out. Counseling is nothing to be ashamed of nor to fear. You owe it to yourself to get help.

Finding a Counselor

From day to day, I, Black Woman, continue to bear the brunt of racism and sexism wherever I go. Oh, to be able to *choose* not to be confronted with one or the other, or both, on any given day—now, that would be the Life.

Who, then, can I turn to when I hurt, real bad? I recall a spiritual that says, "no hidin' place down here." I find myself at therapy's doorstep. Will this counselor usher me to insanity? Because if she does not openly deal with the fact that there is a very low premium on every aspect of my existence, if she does not acknowledge the politics of Black-womanhood, now that would surely drive me nuts.[15]

Eleanor Johnson
"Reflections: On Black Feminist Therapy"

Finding a black counselor or one who has worked with black clients may be difficult. Because of racism, many black therapists, social workers, counselors and psychologists have been steered to working with abused black children, the learning disabled, juvenile offenders and prisoners—where white people thought there would be the most demand for their services and skills. It is only recently that blacks, in sizeable numbers, have begun to use our own therapeutic models based on the black experience instead of those of the white establishment. As a result, many blacks no longer shun mental health service systems, but look to them as a means of maintaining good physical and emotional health.

Probably the best place to start your search for a caring, competent counselor is with other black women friends and co-workers. Ask if they know a local counselor you could see. There are probably community mental health agencies in your area that you can contact. Also check with the YWCA, a battered women's shelter or another women's organization to find out if there is a women's therapy referral service in your community. The therapists who list with a referral service usually offer reduced or sliding-scale fees that allow you to pay for counseling according to your income. Many also grant a free initial interview for you to discuss your issues with the therapist and determine if she is suited to your needs. Check the telephone listings under "mental health," "psychology," "feminist," "women," "battering," and "rape" for information about counseling. You can also call your community crisis line and explain you are looking for a counselor who helps abused women. They may have someone on file who can assist you. Ask your family doctor if s/he can refer you to someone. There will undoubtedly be one counselor somewhere with whom you'll feel comfortable discussing your problems and feelings.

If you are thinking about seeing a male counselor, consider that you have been conditioned to view them as experts and authority figures. Those same views of men as all powerful and all knowing have contributed to society's acceptance of domestic violence.

A black male counselor, although more acceptable racially, may not be sensitive to your position as an abused black woman. He may identify with the attitudes and experiences of the man who is abusing you. He may not be able to listen to you objectively, though as a professional, he should surely try. Because he understands our racial pressures and oppressions, a black male counselor can be as invested in keeping the black family together as you are. He may encourage you to "bear up," "be strong," "keep the faith" or work it out with your partner for the sake of the children and the race. But your counselor does not have to go home and live with an abusive partner like you do. He does not have to worry about how he's going to "keep the faith" while trying to keep the peace too.

A black woman counselor who understands and is sensitive to the issues involved in domestic violence would be ideal. However, if she is not to be found, chances are you will have to consider seeing a white woman counselor.

Regardless of gender or race, the counselor you ultimately choose should treat you professionally. Although some of your experiences might be similar to those of other abused women, your counselor should attempt to get to know you as an individual, rather than offer treatment based on stereotypical views about abused women.

There are certain practices that are generally considered completely unethical. For instance, if your counselor approaches you sexually or does not maintain the confidentiality of your therapeutic relationship, you have every right to leave that counselor and even report the behavior. However, other practices that might also be harmful to you may not be so obvious. A few guidelines can help insure that your counselor does not do additional damage to you because of a lack of understanding of domestic violence or your perspectives as a black woman.

Under no circumstances should you continue to see a counselor who tells you violence is a natural part of black life; who says you provoked your partner; who does not believe you are in serious danger when you say you are; who makes fun of the way you express yourself; who uses any kind of racial slur; who forces you to try counseling techniques that make you uncomfortable; or who suggests you relieve the stress in your life with alcohol, drugs or increased sexual activity.

If you have never had counseling before, locating a counselor and beginning the process of sharing and self-disclosure may "work your last nerve." You may be terrified to talk with a stranger about your problems. You may wonder if you are being judged or if what you say is "right." The key to all your concerns is trust and building a trusting relationship with a counselor does not happen overnight.

Developing trust with your counselor depends on several things: your counselor's skills and techniques, the manner in which you present your problems, your personal commitment to the counseling process, and what you expect to get out of counseling. It may be a good idea to evaluate these issues before you start seeing someone regularly.

The Counseling Process

There will be times when you perhaps feel worse after a session than you did before you talked to your counselor. As one abused woman said, you may leave asking yourself, "I pay money for *this*?" Ironic as it may seem, it is probably when you ask yourself that question that the healing process has begun.

At first, you may only talk to your counselor about "safe" things like your job, family, hobbies or activities you did during the week. However, as the process continues and you begin to trust your counselor you are likely to reveal experiences that really hurt or puzzled you. You may find yourself telling your counselor something you hadn't thought about in years or something you thought was completely unimportant to you. This is because in order to survive in an abusive relationship you have had to steel yourself against really feeling your emotions. You have probably repressed mountains of rage, resentment, shame, helplessness, disgust, and guilt about being abused. As you develop a trusting relationship with your counselor these powerful feelings will start to surface. And when you express your feelings, you'll begin to heal.

Counseling can be a very difficult and emotionally draining process. It can also help you regain your strength and sense of power. Unlike the abuse you have suffered, counseling will not kill you. The key to a successful experience is commitment, caring and trust between you and your counselor.

Support Groups

In addition to, or sometimes instead of individual counseling, you should consider participating in a support group for abused women. A support group provides exactly what the name says — support and encouragement for you from other women who know how you feel and understand what you're talking about. They know your issues because they have been in the same situation you have. They've heard the same promises you have and watched them be broken. They've filed charges like you have and dropped them. They've felt low-down, broke-down and put-down like you have. They've thought about killing him like you have, prayed like you have, wondered if they were losing their minds or if the situation would ever get any better — just like you have. As Juanita found out, joining a support group can end your isolation by putting you in touch with those people you thought didn't exist — other abused black women who have suffered just like you.

> A friend told me about this support group for battered black women and I just didn't want to hear about it. My ears were open, but my mind was shut. I was afraid of what people would think — that they would know I was one of 'them.' But I eventually went — I suppose I was so miserable I knew I had to. And it was hard at first just like I thought it would be. But it was *so* good to see other black faces — to finally talk to other women who'd been in the same situation as me. We laughed, we cried. We talked about everything. It got to the point that those meetings were the highlight of my week. Some of my friends even wanted to go because they saw what a change it made in me. You know, black women can do a lot of things we think we can't do. Like learning we can be somebody without a man. That we don't have to be beaten up, that our kids don't have to be scared to death. That our pride and our families don't have to be ruined.

Support groups for abused women are part of a growing self-help movement in the country. The rationale behind them is that you know more about your life than anyone else and that the best place for you to look for emotional support and practical help is often from other abused women.

Support groups for abused women vary in their size and organizational structure. Some are led by trained counselors who consider domestic violence their field of expertise. Others are run by grassroots activists who have served leadership roles in the women's movement for many years. And there are of course support groups that are organized and led by formerly abused women. The role of the leader or leaders in all cases is to facilitate the exchange of ideas and experiences between abused women.

Battered women's shelters, churches, community centers, or the local YWCA are places where support group meetings are often held. They are usually free and sometimes childcare is provided.

Many support groups have a "drop-in" format meaning that meetings are not mandatory. You can choose to attend whenever you want. Sometimes counselors organize abused women's groups for a specific period of time. In these groups, participants may be asked to pay a fee and are usually expected to attend meetings regularly. Efforts are made in all abused women's groups to insure the safety of participants and to maintain confidentiality.

A support group can be a critical factor in helping you develop or reclaim your self-esteem. The strength and humor you see in other black women as they talk about the lies they've been told and the slaps they've survived will help you see that you also have those qualities. Likewise, seeing other black women cry and express their vulnerabilities can free you to let down your defenses and stop being the "strong black woman."

A support group can help foster feelings of intimacy and trust between black women. For too long we have been told and perhaps too many of us have believed that we will talk about each other, steal each other's men and stab each other in the back whenever we get the chance. These myths have lived long and destructive lives. It is time for black women to put them to rest, or at least begin to talk about them openly.

Being in a support group can give you the courage to stop denying that you are involved with an abusive man and that your life may be in real danger. You can begin to look at your situation objectively and develop approaches to problem-solving that have worked for other black women. For instance, you may never think of using your gardening skills for relaxation, exercise or perhaps to supplement your income until you hear it or something similar mentioned in your support group. Because you have heard for so long that you can't do anything, you may indeed forget all the skills and abilities you have. A support group can be a stimulus for growth, change and a reawakening of yourself. If you see other abused black women making changes in their lives, you'll realize you can do it too—be it following through on prosecution, taking a class, auditioning for a play or going to a movie by yourself. A support group can help you gain a proper perspective on your life. You may have been scared to death, sick to death or almost beaten to death, but in a support group you'll be acknowledged for being a survivor. You'll find much love and support from women who want you to stay alive.

Some facilitators of support groups for abused black women say that it is sometimes difficult to keep the groups active. You may be reluctant to attend meetings because you fear another woman in the group might know your partner or that your confidentiality will not be honored. You may not want to appear ''weak'' in front of other black women.

There is nothing wrong with having these feelings. But you might also consider a support group as a way you can overcome them and learn how to communicate more effectively with other black women. By talking about your fears, you can help shatter some of the cultural myths that have kept black women distant from and suspicious of each other. You can open yourself up to the beauty, wisdom and supportive love of other black women.

Racially Mixed Groups

Your chances of finding a support group specifically for abused black women are best if you live in a large, metropolitan area. However, because blacks are only beginning to address the issue of violence within our communities, not all the resources (human or financial) have been developed that will insure the long-term existence of support groups for abused black women. This means that if you want to connect immediately with other abused women, you may have to attend a racially mixed support group that might be run by a white leader.

Like the abused black woman who sees a white woman counselor for individual therapy, you may bring some suspicions to a racially mixed support group. Because of relationships between white women and black men, you may view white group members symbolically as competitors or threats to your relationships. You may be afraid that the information you share in the support group will be used to perpetuate racist views about black men. You may be reluctant to talk about racism in front of white women or feel the need to always appear strong. In short, you may simply not believe that it is safe for you to discuss your relationship with a black man in a racially mixed group.

Perhaps ''head-on'' is the best way for you to approach this sensitive issue. Share your fears and suspicions with the group leader or individual group members. Ask them to respond to your views. See if they understand your position. Ask them and yourself if it is possible to work through the racial barriers that exist.

Trust your intuition as to whether a racially mixed support group will be helpful or harmful to you. Ask other black women who have participated in such groups to share their experience with you.

Although there may be some added stresses to participating in a racially mixed support group, it can also be a rewarding experience for you. The group can provide an opportunity for you to take a leadership role in initiating discussions about racism and other barriers that exist between women such as class, religion and sexual preference. There is an additional benefit to participating in a racially mixed support group. It will give you living proof that battering crosses all racial and ethnic boundaries. This commonality of experience can and does help abused women understand that oppressive social systems support the violence against all women in our society. It can give you the courage to change your life.

You can get information about support groups from the same sources you contacted about individual counseling—shelters, women's therapy referral services, community mental health agencies and the YWCA.

If you can't find a support group in your community, consider starting one yourself. *Talking It Out* (Resources) is a book with excellent practical and philosophical information about support groups. If "support group" sounds too serious, you can call your group a club or some other name. It is possible for you and other women to share your experiences even if there is no organized support group in your community.

Friends and Family

Because of our extended family system, friends and family often overlap in many black people's lives. Many of us have "play" mothers, fathers, sisters, brothers and cousins who are no blood relation to us, but who may have played a significant role in our upbringing. They are considered as much a part of our family as real aunts, uncles and grandmothers. This support network enriches the black community and nurtures us individually as we face the challenges of daily living. It can, however, serve as a double-edged sword, helping and hurting when we go to family or friends about the violence in our lives.

Couples tend to socialize and build relationships with other couples. Chances are that friends you'd choose to speak with about your partner's abusive behavior are friends of his too. They might have divided loyalties and feel you are pressuring them to take sides about your relationship. Your friends may listen, but really not want to interfere in what they consider to be a personal and private matter between you and your partner. Because they want to believe that you are still the happy couple you may outwardly appear to be, your friends may not take your revelations of abuse seriously. This situation can cause you to think you are crazy or stupid for making a big deal out of something your friends listen to calmly. Or else, it may upset you because it might seem that not even your best and most trusted friends care that you are being abused.

The truth is that neither your family nor friends have been trained to identify or understand all the complex issues involved in domestic violence. They may think it is his job or lack of one, his drinking or his jealousy that is causing your partner to assault you. Because abusive men are sometimes outstanding members of the community, your family and friends may only know your partner as a good father, a committed Little League coach—as a man who always brings the paycheck home. Similarly, they may find it hard to believe that a strong and independent woman like you would put up with abuse and therefore suspect you must be doing something to "deserve it" or that you "like it." Their lack of information and misconceptions about domestic violence can make family and friends ineffective resources to help you stop the violence in your life.

On the opposite end of the spectrum of friends and family members who may not seem to care about your abuse are the people who will jump right in and intervene completely for you. These relatives and friends may insist that you call the police, leave your partner immediately or offer to confront him on your behalf. Occasionally such a response can complicate your situation. For example, your partner may refuse to let people who criticize his behavior come to your house.

Despite their good intentions, a friend or relative who tells you what to do or tries to solve all your problems for you is not being very helpful to you. For like the man who is abusing you, they are denying you the opportunity to take charge of your own life. By not allowing you to decide when and how you wish to deal with the violence in your life, they may undermine your sense of confidence and ability to make independent decisions.

Your family and friends probably care a lot about what is happening to you even though their silences, misconceptions or "take charge" tendencies may not provide exactly the kind of help you need. Unless you and your partner have been exceptionally skillful in hiding the difficulties between you, family and friends probably have some idea that there are problems in your household. In fact, many of the people who phone domestic hotlines for information identify themselves as selves as friends or relatives of women who are being abused.

Within their limitations, your friends and family may be positive and supportive resources. Determine who you can go to for emotional comfort, shelter, a warm meal, peace, quiet financial or childcare assistance if need be. But do not expect any of them to end or completely understand the abuse you suffer.

Support from the Church

Instead of seeking active change in the ''here and now'' some people accept their earthly sufferings and look forward to claiming their reward in heaven. This life, they believe, is a burdensome but necessary cross to bear in order to attain life everlasting. Such is the philosophy of many blacks, who because of our oppression and the failings of mankind, have simply chosen to put our trust in the Lord. The spirituals and gospel songs that are an integral part of the black church, emphasize this theme:

> What a friend we have in Jesus
> All of our sins and griefs to bear
> What a privilege it is to carry
> Everything to God in Prayer.

Throughout our history, the church has held a predominant place in black people's lives. It was a deep, abiding faith in a ''greater good'' and a ''Higher Power'' that gave slave families their spiritual strength and unity. They endured the wrenching pain of losing loved ones on the auction block because they had a firm belief that their families would be reunited in another life.

Although we were freed from slavery, ''freedom'' did not bring blacks total access into American life. Denied participation in political activities and enjoying only limited educational, cultural and economic opportunities, we again turned to the church for support that a racist America did not provide. When restaurant owners, motel managers, school officials and real estate agents bolted their doors against us, the church door was wide open. After being brow-beaten and humiliated by white society we could restore our faith and reclaim a sense of dignity through the teachings and activities of the black church. It is in the church that many of us have developed not only our religious beliefs, but other personal and leadership skills.

Yet religious beliefs or fear of rejection from the church may be keeping you in an oppressive, abusive relationship.

> When he started beating me I went to the elders of the church. They said I couldn't leave because it would be a bad reflection on other church members. I didn't want to bring shame on the rest of the congregation. The church and my faith are very important to me.

If you go to your pastor for help about the violence in your life, you may be told, as the black woman quoted above was, to essentially "love, honor and obey" the man who is abusing you. Your pastor may read scriptures to you that perpetuate male dominance over women. This is not necessarily surprising since the church (black or white) is a male-dominated institution. It is time, however, to begin to challenge those members of the black clergy who are contributing to the continued abuse of black women through their lack of knowledge about domestic violence and/or sexist attitudes.

As with the issues of rape, incest, homosexuality and alcoholism, clergy members are only beginning to receive adequate training on domestic violence. It is only in the past decade or so that many of these issues have lost their social stigmas. Because black women usually comprise seventy percent of any black congregation, it is perhaps more regrettable, but no more surprising that the black clergy has been as uninformed about the extent and severity of domestic violence as anyone else.

Perhaps it has been advantageous for your pastor to minimize the domestic violence within his congregation. Just as you may have denied your partner's abusive behavior to save face, your pastor may use silence and denial to continue the social myth that violence simply does not happen in "good Christian families." To acknowledge domestic violence is to admit, some pastors may think, that the church has failed in its mission. It may reflect poorly on your pastor's word and leadership, because domestic violence clearly indicates that there are some wayward sheep in his flock. Black clergy members, often because of their powerful positions within our communities, may be reluctant to make such admissions.

And so, you may be told to accept and forgive the sins of your abusive partner as Christ did for us when he died on the cross. You pastor may tell you to read Ephesians 5:21, "Wives, submit yourselves unto your own husbands," and urge you to make the sacrifice for your family. You may be told that your abuse is punishment for being spiritually deficient and that if you pray more it will go away. As one abused black woman reported, your paster might even say, "Jesus dropped the charges, so why can't you?"

If your pastor encouraged you to read further in Ephesians you'd find:

> Husbands love your wives, just as Christ loved the church and gave himself up for her to make her holy . . . and to present her to himself as a radiant church, without stain or wrinkle or any other blemish, but holy and blameless. In this same way, husbands ought to love their wives as their own bodies. He who loves his wife loves himself. After all, no one ever hated his own body, but he feeds and cares for it, just as Christ does for the church. (Ephesians 5:25–29)

It is not and never has been God's will that you bow down blindly and accept your partner's abusive behavior. Men who resort to brute force and domination in their relationships deserve strong disapproval and a resounding message that their behavior is wrong from all members of society, including the clergy.

Some church leaders are beginning to confront the real issues of domestic violence and its destructive impact on black families. Some are closely affiliated with shelters for battered women or provide meeting rooms for support groups. But the total strength of the black church as a resource for addressing all aspects of violence in our communities has yet to be tapped. Until such time, it is perhaps best for you to remember that scriptures can be interpreted in many ways and that a family where there is constant upheaval, violence and abuse is not the "holy family" your pastor may urge you to "save."

Perhaps with the support of other black women in your congregation, you can approach your pastor or other church leaders to invite a speaker or sponsor an educational workshop on domestic violence. Try calling a battered women's shelter for suggestions of people in your community who have spoken to church groups about this issue before. Ask friends you might have from other congregations if they've had such programs at their church. Contact the Center for the Prevention of Sexual and Domestic Violence (see Resources). It is an interreligious, educational ministry serving both the religious and secular communities.

The words of black poet Ntozake Shange can provide inspiration when you face situations, like an abusive relationship, that challenge your religion or faith:

> i found god in myself
> & i loved her / i loved her fiercely

Chapter Eight
Yes You Can

You might wonder if it is really possible to learn to nurture yourself and make changes that will free you from an abusive relationship. As Chaka Khan sings, "As strange as it seems, we make our own dreams come true."

To begin the process of ending the violence in your life, it is essential that you tell someone you are being abused. It is impossible to change your situation or for others to help you if you do not admit there is something wrong in your household. As difficult as it may be to accept that your partner is abusing you, you must stop denying or minimizing the reality of your situation. Of course, it is easy to deny painful or unpleasant things if you think you are the cause of them. This is a defense mechanism all humans have. Hopefully, information you have read in this book thus far has helped you understand that you are not responsible for your partner's abusive behavior. As Elaine said, "I finally accepted that this was really his problem and not my fault the day he came home and jumped on me because the store ran out of charcoal. I wasn't going to get beat up everytime he wanted to barbeque."

Your partner must want to change his behavior. He must believe, contrary to what he's learned in society, that he does not have the right to strike you or anyone else because he's a man. He must learn to work out his frustrations about living in a racist society in healthy, productive ways—not by taking his anguish out on you. These may sound like revolutionary suggestions in a society where all young boys are taught to fight back and violence is viewed by many as an acceptable way of dealing with the often brutal injustices of racism. Perhaps it is through such "radical" thoughts and social changes that our tolerance of all forms of violence in American society will end.

Meanwhile, you can put an end to your personal abuse by learning to love yourself in all your dimensions as a black woman. This does not mean you have to abandon your relationship or betray the black race. You can be supportive and understanding of your partner while acknowledging that it is his responsibility to change his abusive behavior. You might discuss setting up a time schedule by which he will enroll in counseling or job training programs to prove he is sincere about changing his life. This does not mean that you are domineering, simply that you believe you deserve a caring, non-abusive relationship.

Taking such action will help rid you of many of the negative stereotypes you have internalized both within and outside of the relationship. The destructive images and action are all around you—black women murdered, black women raped, "fat, lazy and always pregnant" black women in welfare lines. These images are pervasive in our society. They filter in and affect us, no matter how much black pride or self-esteem we tell ourselves we have.

Learn to recognize your own self-hatred. Take an honest assessment of what you do and do not like about yourself and evaluate how much of your feelings are based on white beauty standards or symbols of success. How often do you greet other black women you might pass on the street? Do you bypass blacks in stores, banks or other professional settings because you assume we are less competent in our jobs than whites? Do you seek out the black women in your community who appear to be improving their lives or do you assume they think they're "better" than you? Have you ever considered that other black women might really value having you as a friend? Your honest answers to these questions can give you an indication of what you really think about yourself and other black women. Remember the emotional scars in all of us run deep. They go back as far as our history in this country and none of us will recover from the damage overnight. But we cannot begin to overcome our insecurities or self-hatred until we take an honest look at why these feelings exist.

It is not selfish to nurture yourself as you have nurtured so many others. Go back to school, take a vacation, exercise, pursue the jobs you are really interested in and believe you are qualified to do. So much of our black beauty and abilities have been disguised by poverty, nutritional deficiencies, excessive physical and emotional stress. You can begin to overcome some of these patterns if you start taking even small steps toward a more healthy life like Roz, one abused black woman, did.

I'm not the kind of woman who is ever going to exercise on a regular basis. But I've always wanted to be more physically active. So I decided I'd help my son with his paper route one day a week. I go out with him and help deliver the papers. I enjoy the walking and meeting the people in the neighborhood. My son likes it too because he says having me with him makes it easier to collect the money.

Changing your patterns and your relationship will involve pain, fear and lots of hard work. Some days you may feel lonely, depressed, angry and overwhelmed by it all. You may get sick of calling the police, listening to attorneys or spilling your heart out to a counselor and wondering if any of it is helping at all. You may be tempted to just give up and live with things the way they are.

The police, attorneys, counselors, shelter workers, friends, relatives, etc. are very important resources who can be supportive and help you change the direction of your life. However, none of them have the absolute power to stop your partner from abusing you. Not one of them can do more for you than you can do for yourself, by taking the steps that will make you really believe you deserve a loving, non-abusive relationship.

Like black poet Chirlane McCray, whose poem closes this book, try going to the depths of your being and face every word and deed that has ever hurt you. You'll probably feel pain and shed many tears. But you'll also discover that you can cry and the world will not fall apart. You'll find that you are still a loving, caring, gifted, valuable, unique and beautiful black woman. You are a black woman who deserves to be loved and respected by your partner, as well as the rest of society.

I Used to Think

I used to think
I can't be a poet
because a poem is being everything you can be
in one moment,
speaking with lightning protest
unveiling a fiery intellect
or letting the words drift feather-soft
into the ears of strangers
who will suddenly understand
my beautiful and tortured soul.
But, I've spent my life as a Black girl
a nappy-headed, no-haired,
fat-lipped,
big-bottomed Black girl
and the poem will surely come out wrong
like me.

And, I don't want everyone looking at me.

If I could be a cream-colored lovely
with gypsy curls,
someone's pecan dream and sweet sensation,
I'd be poetry in motion
without saying a word
and wouldn't have to make sense if I did.
If I were beautiful, I could be angry and cute
instead of an evil, pouting mammy bitch
a nigger woman, passed over
conquested and passed over,
a nigger woman
to do it to in the bushes.

My mother tells me
I used to run home crying
that I wanted to be light like my sisters.
She shook her head and told me
there was nothing wrong with my color.

She didn't tell me I was pretty
(so my head wouldn't swell up).

Black girls cannot afford to
have illusions of grandeur,
not ass-kicking, too-loud-laughing,
mean and loose Black girls.

And even though in Afrika
I was mistaken for someone's fine sister or cousin
or neighbor down the way,
even though I swore
never again to walk with my head down,
ashamed,
never to care
that those people who celebrate
the popular brand of beauty
don't see me,
it still matters.

Looking for a job, it matters.
Standing next to my lover
when someone light gets that
"she ain't nothin come home with me" expression
it matters.

But it's not so bad now.
I can laugh about it,
trade stories and write poems
about all those put-downs,
my rage and hiding.
I'm through waiting for minds to change,
the 60's didn't put *me* on a throne
and as many years as I've been
Black like ebony
Black like the night
I have seen in the mirror
and the eyes of my sisters
that pretty is the woman in darkness
who flowers with loving.

Chirlane McCray

Notes

1. Evelyn Reed, *Women's Evolution* (New York: Pathfinder Press, 1975), p. 96.
2. *Aegis: Magazine to End Violence Against Women,* May-June, 1979.
3. Diana Russell, *Sexual Exploitation, Rape, Child Sexual Abuse, Workplace Harassment* (Beverly Hills: Sage, 1984).
4. William A. Stacey and Anson Shupe, *The Family Secret* (Boston: Beacon Press, 1983), pp. 2–3.
5. Inge K. Broverman, et.al., "Sex-Role Stereotypes and Clinical Judgments of Mental Health," *Journal of Consulting and Clinical Psychology,* 34:i., 1970, pp. 1–7.
6. Lenore Walker, *The Battered Woman* (New York: Harper & Row, 1979), pp. 55–70.
7. Zora Neale Hurston, "How It Feels To Be Colored Me," in *I Love Myself When I Am Laughing* (Old Westbury: The Feminist Press, 1978), p. 153.
8. Barbara Smith, introduction to *Home Girls* (New York: Kitchen Table Press, 1983). pp. xxxiv–xxxv.
9. Eleanor Holmes Norton, "Restoring the Traditional Black Family," *New York Times Magazine,* June 2, 1985.
10. Alice Walker, "The Civil Rights Movement: What Good Was It?" in *In Search of Our Mother's Gardens* (New York: Harcourt Brace Jovanovich, 1983), p. 123.
11. Alice Walker, *The Third Life of Grange Copeland* (New York: Harcourt Brace Jovanovich, 1970), p. 55.
12. *New York Times,* May 19, 1985.
13. *Seattle Times,* June 15, 1985.
14. Beth Richie-Bush, "Facing Contradictions: Challenge for Black Feminists," *Aegis,* No. 37, 1983.
15. Eleanor Johnson, "Reflections: On Black Feminist Therapy" in *Conditions Five: The Black Women's Issue,* 1979, p. 113.

Glossary of Terms Used in
Domestic Violence Criminal Cases

Acquitted: Defendant is found not guilty after a trial.

Arraignment: A pre-trial hearing where the defendant answers charges and is told about the rights to have an attorney and a trial.

Bail: A sum of money or surety from the defendant deposited with the court as a promise that if he is released, he will return to court.

Bench trial: A trial where the defendant does not want a jury and has asked only the judge to hear the case and decide if he is guilty.

Bench warrant: An order issued by the court to arrest a defendant usually for failing to appear when ordered.

Calendar: A court calendar lists the trials which will be held each day.

City attorney: The city attorney represents the city and is prosecutor for any violation of the city's criminal ordinances laws.

Civil proceeding: Any court case not a criminal case. May include a petition for divorce, legal separation, or a complaint for damages.

Contempt: Disobeying a court order such as a "no contact order" or the terms of probation may make the defendant guilty of contempt.

Continuance: A delay in a court proceeding until a specific date in the future.

Cross examination: The questions asked of a witness by the opposing attorney during the trial.

Defendant: A person who is charged with a crime.

Defense attorney: The lawyer for the defendant, who may be a Public Defender.

Dismissal: An order of the court withdrawing all criminal charges filed against a defendant.

Evidence: Testimony and objects that help to prove either victim's or suspect's statements.

Eye witness: A person who observed a crime take place.

Hung jury: A jury whose members cannot agree that the defendant is either guilty or not guilty.

Incident report: A report written by the police after responding to a domestic violence call or report written after a victim later reports an incident to the police.

Jury: A group of people from the community who listen to the trial and decide if the defendant is guilty or not guilty.

No contact order: Order issued by a judge directing a defendant to have no contact with you.

Personal recognizance: The release of an arrested person without bail on the promise of a voluntary return to court.

Plea bargain: A deal made by the prosecutor and defense attorney where the defendant agrees to plead guilty to and the prosecutor agrees to recommend a specific sentence.

Pre-sentence report: After a finding of guilty and before sentencing, the defendant may request a pre-sentence report to aid the court in setting a just sentence.

Precinct: In larger cities, the city is broken up into the smaller geographical precincts with a police office or station in each precinct.

Pro bono publico: For the good of the public, free legal representation.

Pro se: A defendant appears pro se if representing him or herself.

Probable cause: Sufficient cause to believe a crime was, or will be committed.

Probation: A judge may order probation as part of a sentence requiring the defendant to perform or not to perform certain action. Probation may include jail time.

Restitution: A court order usually as part of a sentence to reimburse a victim or a shelter for specific costs incurred because of the defendant's actions.

Restraining order: Order issued by a judge during civil proceeding restricting another's contact with you and possibly restricting other conduct also.

Revocation hearing: A hearing to determine if a defendant's release from jail on specific conditions (bail, personal recognizance, probation) should be revoked and the defendant reincarcerated.

Sentencing: A legal process where the defendant hears what the punishment will be.

Stay: A delay in court proceeding until a date to be set in the future.

Submit a case on the record: Judge bases finding of defendant's guilt or innocence on a reading of the police report with no testimony or witnesses.

Subpoena: The legal paper that commands a witness to appear in court.

Suspect: A person who is believed to have committed a crime.

Testimony: Statements made in court by a person under oath.

Verdict: The decision that a jury or judge reaches at the conclusion of a trial determining the guilt or innocence of the defendant.

Suggested Reading and Resources

The following selected list is for abused black women as well as for all individuals working to help women end abusive relationships.

Domestic Violence

Fortune, Marie and Denise Hormann, *Family Violence: A Workshop Manual for Clergy and Other Service Providers*. Seattle: The Center for the Prevention of Sexual and Domestic Violence (1914 N. 34th, #205, Seattle, WA 98103), 1980.

Martin, Del. *Battered Wives*. Revised edition. San Francisco: Volcano Press (Dept. B, 330 Ellis St., San Francisco, CA 94102), 1981.

McNulty, Faith. *The Burning Bed: The True Story of an Abused Wife*. New York: Bantam Books, 1981.

NiCarthy, Ginny. *Getting Free: A Handbook for Women in Abusive Relationships*. Seattle: Seal Press, 1982.

NiCarthy, Ginny, Karen Merriam and Sandra Coffman. *Talking It Out: A Guide to Groups for Abused Women*. Seattle: Seal Press, 1984.

Paris, Susan. *Mommy and Daddy Are Fighting* (a book for children about domestic violence). Seattle: Seal Press, 1985.

Schechter, Susan. *Women and Male Violence: The Visions and Struggles of the Battered Women's Movement*. Boston: South End Press, 1982.

Walker, Lenore E. *The Battered Woman*. New York: Harper & Row, 1979.

Warrior, Betsy. *Battered Women's Directory (eighth edition)*. Cambridge: Betsy Warrior (46 Pleasant St., Cambridge, MA 02139), 1982.

Zambrano, Myrna M. *Mejor Sola Que Mal Acompañada: Para la Mujer Golpeada/For the Latina in an Abusive Relationship*. Seattle: Seal Press, 1985.

Black Women

Angelou, Maya. *I Know Why the Caged Bird Sings*. New York: Random House, 1970.

Gather Together in My Name. New York: Random House, 1974.

Singing and Swinging and Getting Merry Like Christmas. New York: Random House, 1976.

Heart of a Woman. New York: Random House, 1981.

Shaker, Why Don't You Sing? New York: Random House, 1983.

Bambara, Toni Cade. *Gorilla, My Love*. New York: Random House, 1972.

The Salt Eaters. New York: Random House, 1980.

Cliff, Michelle. *Claiming an Identity They Taught Me to Despise*. Watertown, MA: Persephone Press, 1981.

Abeng. Trumansburg, NY: The Crossing Press, 1984.

Cochran, Jo, J.T. Stewart and Mayumi Tsutakawa, eds. *Gathering Ground: New Writing and Art by Northwest Women of Color*. Seattle: Seal Press, 1984.

Cooper, J. California. *A Piece of Mine*. Navarro, CA: Wild Trees Press (PO Box 378, Navarro, CA 95463), 1984.

Evans, Mari, ed. *Black Women Writers (1950–1980)*. Garden City: Anchor/Doubleday, 1984.

Hull, Gloria, et.al. *But Some of Us Are Brave: Black Women's Studies*. Old Westbury, NY: The Feminist Press, 1981.

Hurston, Zora Neale. *Their Eyes Were Watching God*. Champaign IL: University of Illinois Press, 1978.

I Love Myself When I Am Laughing . . . & Then When I Am Looking Mean & Impressive. Old Westbury NY: The Feminist Press, 1979.

Kincaid, Jamaica. *Annie John*. New York: Farrar, Straus, Giroux, 1985.

Lorde, Audre. *Chosen Poems: Old and New*. New York: Norton, 1982.

Zami, A New Spelling of My Name. Trumansburg NY: The Crossing Press, 1983.

Sister Outsider. Trumansburg NY: The Crossing Press, 1984.

Marshall, Paule. *Brown Girl Brownstones*. Old Westbury NY: The Feminist Press, 1981.

Praisesong for the Widow. New York: G.P. Putnam's Sons, 1983.

Moraga, Cherríe and Gloria Anzaldúa, eds. *This Bridge Called My Back: Writings by Radical Women of Color*. New York: Kitchen Table Women of Color Press (PO Box 2753, Rockefeller St. New York NY 10185), 1981.

Morrison, Toni. *The Bluest Eye*. New York: Washington Square Press, 1972.

Sula. New York: Knopf, 1973.

Naylor, Gloria. *The Women of Brewster Place*. New York: Viking, 1982.

Linden Hills. New York: Ticknor & Fields, 1985.

Parker, Pat. *Movement in Black*. Trumansburg NY: The Crossing Press, 1983.

Jonestown & Other Madness. Ithaca NY: Firebrand Books, 1985.

Shange, Ntozake. *For Colored Girls Who Have Considered Suicide When the Rainbow Is Enuf*. New York: Macmillan, 1977.

Sassafras, Cypress and Indigo. New York: St. Martin's Press, 1982.

Betsey Brown. New York: St. Martin's Press, 1985.

Smith, Barbara. *Home Girls: A Black Feminist Anthology*. New York: Kitchen Table, 1983.

Walker, Alice. *The Third Life of Grange Copeland*. New York: Harcourt, Brace, Jovanovich, 1970.

In Love and Trouble. New York: HBJ, 1974.

Meridian. New York: HBJ, 1976.

You Can't Keep A Good Woman Down. New York: HBJ, 1982.

The Color Purple. New York: HBJ, 1982.

In Search of Our Mothers' Gardens. New York: HBJ, 1983.

Walker, Margaret. *Jubilee*. New York: Houghton Mifflin, 1966.

Periodicals

Essence, a monthly magazine for black women, 1500 Broadway, New York NY 10036

SAGE: A Scholarly Journal About Black Women, P.O. Box 42741, Atlanta GA 30311-0741

Between Ourselves: Women of Color Newspaper, P.O. Box 1939, Washington D.C. 20013

Aegis: Magazine on Ending Violence Against Women, P.O. Box 21033, Washington D.C. 20009

Organizations

National Coalition Against Domestic Violence. 1500 Massachusetts Ave NW, Suite 35, Washington D.C. 20005

Black Women's Health Project, 450 Auburn Ave N.E., Suite 157, Atlanta GA 30312

National Clearinghouse on Domestic Violence, P.O. Box 2309, Rockville MD 20852

Resource Center on Family Violence/ Center for Women Policy Studies, 2000 P St. NW, Suite 508, Washington D.C. 20036

The Center for the Prevention of Sexual and Domestic Violence, 1914 N. 34th, Seattle WA 98103

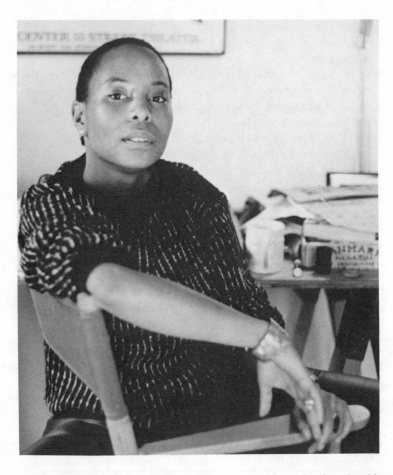

photo: Candace Coughlin

Author's Note: Evelyn C. White is a former advocate for the Seattle City Attorney's Family Violence Project. She grew up in Gary, Indiana and currently lives in New York where she writes on a variety of black, feminist and cultural issues.

Chain Chain

"*Some days you may be absolutely convinced that you will not stay another minute. Other days you may not be able to imagine life without him.*"

It's not easy to make the decision to stay or leave, but this book can help. *Chain Chain Change* is for the black woman who wants to understand the role of emotional abuse and violence in her life, and for the activist and professional who works with domestic violence. *Chain Chain Change* discusses stereotypes and cultural assumptions and offers positive suggestions on getting support from emergency agencies, the legal system, shelters, counselors and the church. *Chain Chain Change* is for any black woman who has ever wondered if she's abused—for any black woman who wants to turn her life around.

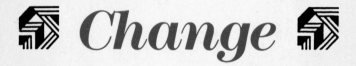 # Change

"*Chain Chain Change* looks at the experience of being abused within the context of black culture, revealing a fresh, a more colorful perspective. In doing so, the author offers black abused women gentle guidance, respectful advice and a strong sense of hope, as well as information that is sound, accurate and realistic. The book's step-by-step approach makes the process of reaching out for help much easier. For battered women advocates, *Chain Chain Change* exposes the cultural and institutional barriers black women face and offers an opportunity for a new understanding of our life experiences. This is an important contribution to the battered women's movement; it is, to quote Evelyn C. White '. . . an opportunity to open ourselves up to the beauty, wisdom and supportive love of black women.'"

—Beth Richie-Bush, MSW
Co-chair, National Coalition Against Domestic Violence
    Women of Color Task Force
Director of Social Services
    East Harlem Council of Human Services

$4.95   The Seal Press   ISBN: 0-931188-25-3